Anatomy and Kinesiology
for Ballet Teachers

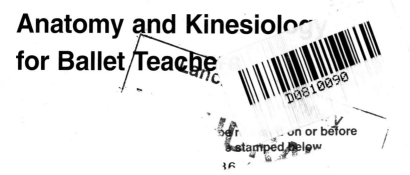

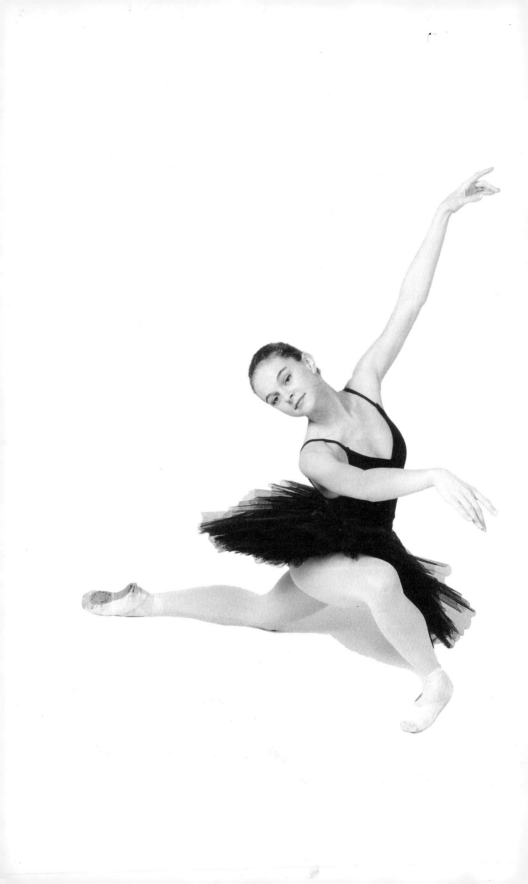

Anatomy and Kinesiology for Ballet Teachers

Eivind Thomasen
Rachel-Anne Rist

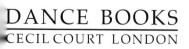

DANCE BOOKS
CECIL COURT LONDON

Po 01471

201.198.

Published in 1996 by Dance Books Ltd
15 Cecil Court, London WC2N 4EZ

Copyright © Eivind Thomasen, Rachel-Anne Rist 1996

ISBN 1 85273 048 X

A CIP catalogue record for this book
is available from the British Library

Photographs by Mike Bass, Lime Tree Studios, Tring
Illustrations by Katie Butt
Design by Sanjoy Roy

Printed and bound in Great Britain by
H. Charlesworth & Co. Ltd, Huddersfield

Contents

Foreword

I am delighted that Eivind Thomasen's manuscript, left with me and my husband when he last visited London, has been, with the permission of his family, carefully and succinctly edited by Rachel Rist, for the express reason of helping dancers and teachers to understand more about the basic anatomy of the dancer's body.

Professor Thomasen, who was Consultant to the Royal Danish Ballet, and known to dancers and surgeons the world over, was the son of a blacksmith and an extraordinary man. He was totally dedicated to his work and to helping others, particularly dancers, for whom he had a great affinity.

He was an innovator with a vast knowledge of human anatomy, and also had a great interest in equine injuries; and he had been a forerunner in working with polio sufferers at the famous Orthopaedic Hospital at Aarhus in Denmark.

My deepest impressions were not only of a brilliant diagnostician and surgeon, but also of a man who was a true Christian, ever mindful of his family and of those with whom he came into contact.

Dame Merle Park, DBE
Director, The Royal Ballet School

Preface

In writing an anatomy and kinesiology book for dance teachers, decisions have been made to keep the information as relevant as possible. The subjects are vast, and there are many excellent reference books which will go into much more detail than is presented here. My criteria have been the inclusion of information that teachers of dance should have. Much has been left out, and much has been greatly simplified.

I have retained the original title of the book as written by Professor Thomasen; although it refers to ballet teachers, teachers of contemporary and jazz techniques of dance should not feel excluded. Most of the information in this book is relevant to anyone who teaches dance.

Permission to use Professor Thomasen's manuscript as the basis for the book has been kindly given by his relatives. I am much indebted to them, and in particular to his daughter, Sigrid Clerk.

I would like to thank my husband, Alastair Greetham MCSP, for his excellent help and advice in preparing this book. All anatomy and kinesiology has been checked by him, and I am indebted to him for much teaching along the way.

Rachel-Anne Rist, MA
January 1995

viii

Introduction

The demands of classical ballet dictate that the whole body should function perfectly, in particular the vertebral column and the limbs.

A knowledge of anatomy and the functions of joints and muscles is important for ballet teachers who select and train ballet students, and it is also of value to the teachers who train professional dancers.

The knowledge of how the vertebral column and the limbs are constructed, and of their functions, is of vital importance for dance teachers, as it enables efficient use of the body and the avoidance of unnecessary strain.
Professor Eivind Thomasen

Professor Thomasen left a rough first draft of this manuscript with Dame Merle Park. He had probably intended to work on it and then publish it as a companion to his excellent book *Diseases and Injuries of Ballet Dancers*. Unfortunately Professor Thomasen died before he was able to complete the work. I knew Eivind Thomasen, as he had twice operated on me successfully. It would be fair to say that through his work he inspired me to learn and understand the dancer's body.

Working from someone else's manuscript is a huge responsibility. The draft he left behind was very rough, and difficult to understand as he was writing in his second language. I realised that much basic anatomy had been assumed, and so where possible I have included simple descriptions and 'translated' the anatomy for a dance teacher as far as possible, without deviating too much from Thomasen's ideas. I have also greatly extended the book so as to make it as comprehensive as possible for those students and teachers who are learning anatomy for dance teaching examinations.

To those teachers who look through the book and are intimidated by names and detailed anatomical descriptions – courage! It is not necessary to learn all the names of muscles and bones. But it is important to understand how the body grows, how it works and how it responds to stress. Training dancers is a huge responsibility, and an essential step is to learn about the body from the inside out. It is a fascinating subject, and as you learn you will become full of admiration for the body, in particular the dancer's body.

I hope Professor Thomasen would have approved of the final book.
Rachel-Anne Rist, MA

Dance requires a unique synthesis of the science of human motion with the art of dance ... conscious awareness of the science of motion can do much to facilitate excellence in performance and prevent injury. The science of human motion provides the dancer with essential information about the structure, function, and achievement of optimal performance.

The merging of art and science is essential in dance.

Sally Sevey Fitt
Dance Kinesiology, 1988

Part 1

The Systems

Terminology

Correct terminology is important in the understanding of anatomy, as it enables the correct identification of the position, location and action of a structure. Anatomical terms, like dance terms and names of steps, provide a vocabulary. They are important to understand as they enable dance teachers to be able to communicate effectively with dance therapists and with medically trained people. It also indicates a knowledge and understanding of anatomy. Terms are very precise, and are also relative to each other and to the surrounding structures. Try to become familiar with these terms and relate them to movements. Correct terms will be used throughout the book – so if in doubt about the meaning of a word, refer back to this glossary until you are familiar with the term.

The anatomical position that is the basis for this terminology is that of a person standing in an upright position, facing forwards, with the palms of the hands facing the front (Fig. 1).

Words which describe position

Anterior	Front, or in front
Posterior	Back, or behind
Medial	Towards the mid-line of the body
Lateral	Away from the mid-line of the body
Proximal	Close to the centre of the body
Distal	Close to the extremity of the body
Superficial	Near the skin surface layer
Deep	Below the superficial layer
Superior	Nearer the top of the body
Inferior	Further away from the top of the body

Words which describe movement

Flexion	An increase in the angle of a joint
Extension	A stretch, or decrease in the angle of a joint
Adduction	Movement towards the mid-line of the body
Abduction	Movement away from the mid-line of the body
Circumduction	The circular range of movement found at a ball-and-socket joint

2

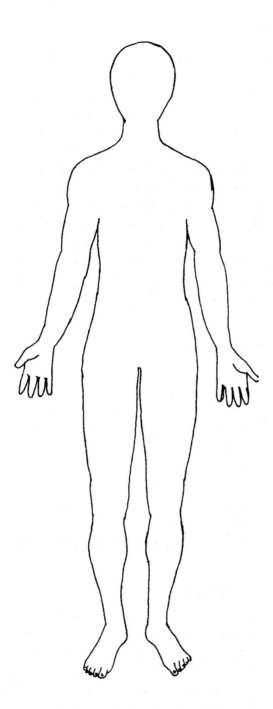

Fig. 1. The basic anatomical position.

Inverted	Sickling inwards
Everted	Sickling outwards
Plantar flexion	Pointing the foot
Dorsiflexion	Extending the ankle or toe joints (known to dancers as flexing the foot upwards)
Pronation	Facing downwards (of the foot or arm)
Supination	Palm upwards, or rolling of ankle or sole upwards
Rotation	The movement of a joint which can rotate, or twist in a certain plane

Words which describe bony features

Apophysis	A bony outgrowth
Condyle	A rounded projection at the end of a bone
Diaphysis	The shaft of a long bone
Epiphysis	The end of a long bone
Exostoses	A bony growth
Foramen	A hole in a bone
Fossa	A hollow depression in a bone
Trochanter	A large bump on a bone
Tubercle	A small bump on a bone
Tuberosity	A bump on a bone

Other anatomical terminology

Atrophy	Muscle wasting or thinning of the body
Collagen	A bundle of fibres formed from a protein. Collagen fibres are found in connective tissue
Connective tissue	Tissue that binds and supports other body tissues (e.g. bone, cartilage, fibrous tissue)
Contusion	A bruise or damage to the tissue without the skin being broken
Effusion	The escape of fluids; a swelling
Fascia	A fibrous connective tissue that may vary in thickness
Haematoma	A swelling of blood
Hyaline cartilage	A special cartilage found on the surface of articulating bones. It is translucent and pearly in appearance
Kinesiology	The science of movement

Lesion	A wound or injury that causes damage to tissues
Myofibril	A strand of muscle tissue
Sprain	A sudden traumatic injury often causing a tear or damage in ligaments.
Strain	Damage to tendons or muscles often caused by overuse of muscular effort

Basic structures and classifications

In order for this book to be as accessible as possible it is necessary to have some understanding of very basic anatomical information and terminology. From the following lists and classifications it should be possible to read this book with some of the key information already understood.

The tissues of the body

The body is composed primarily of cells, which are the basic units of life. Cells form all the structures and organs of the body, and have specialised functions depending on where they are found.

The cells are composed into four basic tissues:

- *Epithelial tissue*. This mainly forms internal and external coverings, for example the skin and the lungs. The purpose of epithelial tissue is mostly protective.
- *Connective tissue*. Confusingly, this is a general term for a type of tissue found in the body, *and* a specific term for a supporting tissue. Connective tissue (general term) comprises cartilage, bone and fibrous connective tissue (specific term). Connective tissue (general term) consists of a matrix of supporting tissue that may be liquid (e.g. blood), solid (e.g. bone), or gelatinous (e.g. cartilage). Types of connective tissue include:

Areolar tissue.	Found almost everywhere in the body connecting one part of the body with another.
Adipose tissue	Consists of fat cells; used for storage of energy, protection and insulation around the body.
Fibrous tissue	Dense collagen fibres; ligaments, tendons, fascia, etc.
Elastic tissue	Where a specific shape is required; e.g. ears, trachea. It is very flexible and often yellow in colour.
Lymphoid tissue	Found in the lymphatic systems.
Cartilage	Found in many areas of the body; has many elastic fibres

- *Muscle tissue.* There are three types of muscle tissue: skeletal, voluntary and cardiac.
- *Nervous tissue.* The types of cells that are used in the nervous system.

We will now look in more detail at the connective tissues with which we are more familiar, and are especially useful in the study of dancers' movements: bone, muscle, tendons, ligaments and cartilage.

What is bone?

Bone is a living substance mostly made up of calcium phosphate and mineral salts. It has a good blood supply via the periosteum, a thin membrane that covers it.

Bone classifications:

Long bones	e.g. femur (thigh bone), tibia (shin bone)
Short bones	e.g. cuboid (foot bone), carpal bone (wrist)
Irregular bones	e.g. ilium (hip bone), vertebra (back bone)
Sesamoid bones	e.g. patella (knee cap), sesamoid bone in foot
Flat bones	e.g. scapula (shoulder blade), skull bones

Bone types:
Cancellous bone has a 'spongy' appearance with tiny holes in, called trabeculae. It is often found in irregular bones.
Compact bone has a smooth appearance with an ivory-like feel. It is found on the surface of most bones.

What is muscle?

Muscles have three properties:

- Extensibility, the ability to lengthen
- Conductivity, the ability to send and receive messages
- Contractility, the ability to contract and shorten

Muscles function with oxygen and energy from a good blood supply.

The waste products of a working muscle included lactic acid, carbon dioxide and heat.

There are two types of muscle fibres:
- Fast twitch or pale fibres, which give quick, explosive movements (used, for example, in a sprint).
- Slow twitch or red fibres, which give slower, aerobic movements (used, for example, in a marathon run). Slow twitch fibres are usually associated with postural muscles.

Dancers use a combination of both types of fibres.

What is a tendon?

A tendon attaches a muscle to a bone. It has flexibility, but is inelastic longitudinally, and very tough. It has very dense collagen fibres. A large flat tendon which spreads the origin of a muscle over a large area is called an aponeurosis. It is extremely rare to change the length of a tendon, but it is often possible to stretch the muscle to which the tendon is attached. Tendons have great strength, but exposed to great force can be damaged and may either rupture or break away from the bony attachment.

What is a ligament?

A ligament guides the movement of a joint, and maintains skeletal structure. It reinforces a joint structure and supports the plane of movement of the joint. It usually attaches bone to bone. Ligaments are inelastic and if permanently overstretched are not able to return to their original length.

What is cartilage?

Cartilage is dense tissue. Bones are initially cartilaginous until growth is completed. There are three types of cartilage:

- Articular hyaline cartilage, found at the end of bones

- White fibrocartilage, with very dense collagen fibres, providing great strength
- Yellow fibrocartilage, a fairly elastic tissue found in the ears, larynx, trachea, nose, etc.

* * *

With a basic understanding of the tissues of the body, each structure necessary for movement will now be examined at a deeper level. Take time to make sure that you understand each section before proceeding in order to build up slowly an understanding of general anatomy.

Bone

Bone functions:
- To provide a structure for the body
- To provide attachments for muscles
- To serve as a reservoir for mineral salts
- To manufacture red blood cells

Inside long bones the medullary cavity contains blood vessels and special cells which produce the red blood cells. In adults the bone marrow consists mostly of fat cells and yellow marrow. Red marrow can be found in the cavities of other shapes of bones.

The development of bone

Bone is a hard, calcified, living tissue. The skeleton in the spine and limbs is developed from cartilage, which is a firm elastic tissue of translucent colour. Cartilage occurs in two forms: temporary cartilage and permanent cartilage. In the foetus the main parts of the skeleton start as temporary cartilage. At birth the skeleton begins ossification by gradual infiltration of mineral salts, and becomes bone. (It is because temporary cartilage changes its character and hardens into bone that it is called 'temporary'.) The second form, permanent cartilage, can be found covering the articulating surfaces of bones, attaching the ribs to the sternum, in the nose, trachea, larynx and between some joints. It always retains its original character.

Temporary cartilage has the ability to grow and be transformed into bone tissue. By the time the child is born, the long bones will have ceased to be made entirely of temporary cartilage. Growth takes place in three places: in the diaphysis and in the two epiphyses. The diaphysis of the bone changes into hard bone by the infiltration of calcium salts. At birth the ends of the long bone (the epiphyses) still consist of temporary cartilage. After birth this temporary cartilage at the end of the long bones continues to grow in all directions, but especially in the direction of the diaphysis of the bone, which has already ossified. The shaft then begins to thicken as new bone is formed on the outside, while in the centre of the bone the tissue disappears, creating a cavity. The solid shaft has now changed into a tube. This cavity is called the medullary cavity, and houses the bone marrow (Fig. 2).

The whole process of the formation of new bone material on the outside and the hollowing out of the centre of the bone shaft is caused by special cells in the bone substance. The bone-building cells are called osteoblasts. The cells that form the cavity are called osteoclasts.

Bone at the hard centre of the diaphysis is smooth in appearance and is typical of the type of bone called compact bone. Bone on the epiphysis (or 'knuckle' of a long bone) has a different appearance. It is full of tiny holes and is sponge-like in appearance. This is called cancellous bone. The tiny holes are called trabeculae, and give strength without adding weight to the massive structure. The internal construction of the trabeculae is such that they are able to offer great support to the limbs, and are laid down along stress lines of the bone. Compact bone often covers the shaft of long bones and lies on top of cancellous bone.

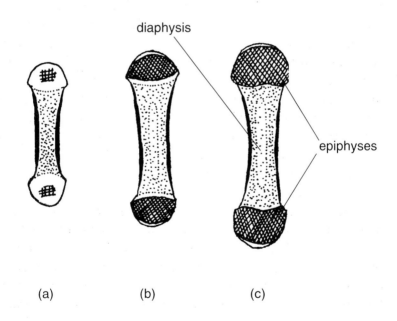

Fig. 2. The growth of a long bone: (a) initial rod of cartilage in shape of bone; (b) ossification begins in the diaphysis and the epiphyses; (c) the two centres of ossification grow towards each other, leaving a line of cartilage at the epiphyseal plate. The centre of the bone begins to become hollow.

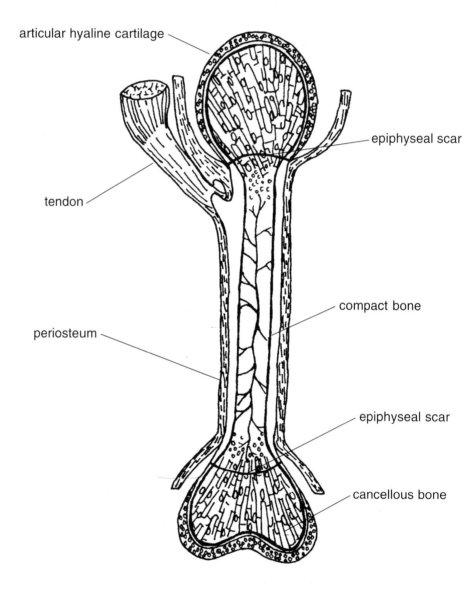

articular hyaline cartilage

epiphyseal scar

tendon

compact bone

periosteum

epiphyseal scar

cancellous bone

Fig. 3. A typical adult long bone.

Between the epiphysis and the diaphysis of the long bone is a layer of cartilage called the epiphyseal plate. This is where growth in length takes place by the transformation of cartilage into bone tissue. This line of cartilage becomes thinner as the bone continues to grow. On X-rays it can be seen as a clear line between the diaphysis and the epiphysis. The epiphyseal plate finally disappears when growth has come to an end and there is solid bone between the two sections.

The process of destruction and reformation of bone substances continues throughout life, even after the skeleton has stopped growing. Bone is living tissue and able to repair itself. In children, bone is able to grow in its normal pattern and able to correct a deformity such as a fracture. However, it responds to its environment and if great pressure in put on a bone, it will protect itself by growing more bone. A good example of this is the enlarged bunion (hallux valgus) often formed by incorrect weight placement on the foot. Because of this ability of bone to adapt to its environment, pointe work should not be commenced until there is strong support in postural muscles and lower leg muscles. It is therefore important to understand the correct distribution of force evenly through the structures of the body.

The growth of the skeleton continues until the age of 14–16 for girls and 16–18 for boys. Some bones do not completely ossify until the age of 24–25.

The structure of bone

The surfaces of bone are covered by a layer of dense fibrous tissue called the periosteum. This is fixed to the bone by collagen fibres. It surrounds the bone except for those areas covered by articular (hyaline) cartilage. The periosteum contains osteoblasts, osteoclasts, blood vessels and nerves (Fig. 3).

Inside compact bone are many tiny cylindrical canals called the Haversian canals. These canals each contain concentric layers (lamellae, flat 'plates' of bone) which run along the length of the bone. The lamellae are arranged according to where stress occurs in a bone. It is believed that arteries and veins found in the periosteum are connected with vessels in the Haversian canals, which are themselves intricately interconnected.

Ability to repair

When a bone is fractured the periosteum is ruptured and blood seeps from the blood vessels into the muscles around the site of the fracture. This is called a haematoma. Connective tissue is formed from the periosteum to the haematoma and from this connection osteoblasts form new bone called callus. This is initially soft, but gradually calcifies and hardens until the fracture is healed and the bone is solid.

Problems associated with growth

- At the epiphyseal plate an active adolescent can sometimes experience pain, especially at the knee. This is commonly called 'growing pain'. During this time it may be necessary to limit the amount of activity especially weight-bearing activities.
- As the epiphyseal plate is still essentially cartilaginous, it is a weak part of the bone. The connection between the diaphysis and the epiphysis may be disrupted by trauma, such as a fracture, after an accident. Such a fracture of the epiphyseal plate may cause a growth disturbance with subsequent deformity at the end of the bone.
- In adolescence the hip may be susceptible to damage at the head of the femur (the long thigh bone). This may slide backwards and downwards due to changes in growth of the epiphyseal plate between the head of the femur and the neck of the femur with a resulting deformity of the hip joint. This may be misdiagnosed, as the adolescent may complain of pain in the knee and not in the hip. It is important to treat this condition as soon as possible to prevent any further sliding of the head of the femur. The head may dislocate completely from the neck, and such a total disruption of the epiphyseal area may end in dead bone in the head of the femur with severe deformity in the hip.
- During the latter part of growth there are some vulnerable areas on the developing bone which are still cartilage. Prominent parts of the skeleton – such as the elbow, the tibial tuberosity (a small lump on the upper end of the shin bone), and the prominent end of the heel bone (the calcaneus) – may be subject to stress in the area of the epiphysis. On these apophyses (a swelling, or outgrowth on the bone) are fixed thick tendons with muscle attachments. Students doing a lot of activity during growth may use powerful movements from muscles that

are anchored by tendons on the epiphyseal plate. There may be pain and tenderness on the apophysis. On the elbow this could be 'tennis elbow'. On the knee this is called 'Schlatter's disease', and on the heel it is called 'Haglund's disease'. The problem will disappear at the end of the growth period, but may cause disruption to training for several months. It is essential to rest during this period, and cease weight-bearing activities which may exacerbate any damage to the epiphyses.

*   *   *

We are able to perform a wide range of movements because of the special juxtaposition of two bones. The bones of the skeleton are linked together to form joints.

Joints

A joint is a connection between bones, and allows some, or little movement. A joint is called an articulation. There are three types of joints:
synovial joints, cartilaginous joints and fibrous joints.

Synovial joints

A synovial joint is characterised by having a wide range of movement. It
may be a ball-and-socket joint (shoulder and hip), a hinge joint (knee and
elbow), or a saddle joint (the ankle). There are other classifications of
synovial joints such as plane, ellipsoid and pivotal. The mobility of the
joint depends on the shape of the reciprocal joint surfaces (Fig. 4).

- *Joint capsule*. The joint cavity between two surfaces is enclosed with a
  joint capsule acting like a cuff from one bone to another. The fibrous
  capsule keeps the two bones together. It is composed of fibrous tissue
  of varying thickness and strength. In hinge joints the capsule is tight
  and strong on the sides but weak and lax in front and back. Supportive structures of fibrous tissue called ligaments help bind the joint
  together and guide the plane of movement. If a joint is sprained the
  fibrous capsule and the ligaments may be ruptured. If the ligaments
  are ruptured the stability of the joint is lost, greatly impairing the joint
  function. The fibrous capsule of the shoulder joint is very lax all
  round to permit great mobility. In the hip joint the fibrous capsule is
  very thick in front with a very strong iliofemoral ligament from the
  upper rim of the socket (acetabulum) to the front of the neck of the
  femur. This ligament limits extension of the joint (backwards movement). Thus the shoulder joint has great mobility and little stability
  and the hip joint has great stability and less mobility.
- *Synovial fluid*. Inside the fibrous capsule is a fine membrane of connective tissue called the synovium. It arises between the two bones from
  the margin of the joint cartilage to the inside of the fibrous capsule. It
  contains blood vessels and nerves. Lining this capsule is the synovial
  membrane, which produces a clear viscous liquid called synovial
  fluid. This lubricates the joint cartilages and nourishes the articular
  surfaces. Synovial fluid allows friction-free movement between the

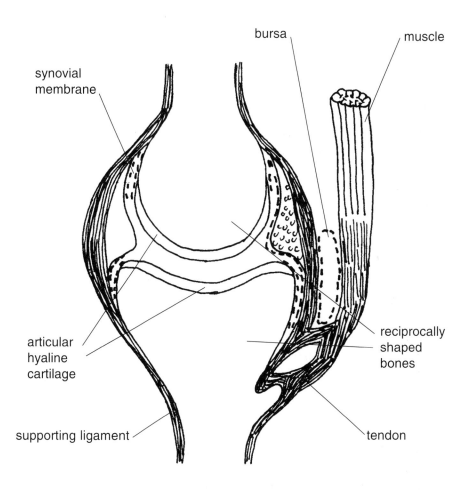

Fig. 4. A typical synovial joint showing reciprocally shaped articulating surfaces covered in hyaline cartilage.

two bone surfaces. If there is damage to the joint it becomes inflamed, causing the synovium to produce more synovial fluid, and the resultant effusion dilates the joint capsule. A mechanical disturbance in a joint such as a free-floating body or a meniscus tear may cause an irritation of the synovial membrane which will produce large amounts of synovial fluid and cause swelling. In cases of severe inflammation in the synovial membrane the joint cartilage may be destroyed resulting in severe pain upon movement. Such inflammation is found in rheumatoid arthritis and infectious arthritis.

- *Bursae.* A bursa is a small sac containing synovial fluid. It is found between two surfaces where friction-free movement is required: between bone and tendon, tendon and tendon, tendon and ligament, or tendon and skin. Its function is to protect from wear and tear. Most synovial joints have several bursae to allow ranges of movement. If a joint is subject to repeated trauma, such as kneeling down, the bursa may swell and become inflamed. This condition is known as bursitis. Bursitis in the knee is known as 'housemaid's knee'; it is more common in jazz dancers who may subject the knee to direct trauma.

- *Articular cartilage.* In synovial joints the ends of two articulating bones are covered with a special cartilage called articular hyaline cartilage. This gives a smooth surface to the bone and is a remnant of the foetal cartilage. The articular cartilage is fixed to the underlying bone, the epiphyseal bone or the short bone. While the bone is growing there is also growth in this cartilage. Articular hyaline cartilage is a living tissue and grows by multiplication of the cells within the cartilage. There are no blood vessels or nerves in the cartilage, but they are present in the bone beneath the cartilage. The source of energy for the living cartilage is synovial fluid. The layer of cartilage is of variable thickness. In the large weight-bearing joints of adults it is about 3–4 mm, but in children where the bone is not yet fully formed around the epiphysis the cartilage is thicker.

  In elderly people the joint cartilage may show some degenerative changes and become thinner. The process of degeneration continues as the thin cartilage may be compressed by the hard bone surfaces, which may themselves deform. At the edges of such degenerated bones there may be bone spurs called osteophytes. Such a joint disease is called osteoarthrosis. Small particles of degenerated joint cartilage are worn away and become loose bodies within the joint cavity.

The result is painful movement with limited mobility and extra production of synovial fluid and thickening of the chronically inflamed membrane.

When a joint has reached its maximum position of stability it is said to be in the 'close packed position'. The two articulating surfaces are fitted as close as possible to each other and the joint is 'locked'. Such an extreme position requires muscular effort to achieve, and is much used by dancers.

Cartilaginous joints

While synovial joints may be called 'freely' movable, cartilaginous joints may be called 'slightly' movable. Some joints consist of a solid connection with fibrocartilaginous tissue and have little movement. An example of this is the joint between two bodies of the vertebrae in the spine. A similar type of joint is found between the two pubic bones at the front of the pelvic, ring called the pubic symphysis.

Fibrous joints

Fibrous joints are immovable and bind two bones firmly together. Examples are the joints between the bones of the skull, and the joints between the tibia and the fibula at both the upper and lower ends where they meet.

*   *   *

The body has articulations that can provide very little, some, or a lot of movement, depending on what type of joint exists between two bones. In order to effect a movement for a joint, an outside force is needed; this is provided by the muscles.

Muscles

There are three kinds of muscles: skeletal muscle (also called voluntary, or striated muscle), cardiac muscle, and smooth muscle (also called involuntary or non-striated muscle). Cardiac muscle is found in the heart, and smooth muscle is mostly found in the digestive system, bladder, etc., and not directly under voluntary control. This section will deal with skeletal muscle.

Structure

Skeletal muscle has three important properties: contractility (the ability to shorten); conductivity (the ability to receive and send impulses or messages); and extensibility (the ability to lengthen). The connective tissue in the muscles around the muscle fibres is fairly dense. Stretching of connective tissue may allow an elongation of the muscle. This extensibility is best obtainable in children before the connective tissue becomes too resistant to extensibility. Unlike tendons, muscles do have the capacity to be stretched.

A muscle is a collection of fibres, each of which is an individual muscle cell. Through a microscope it is possible to see that the single muscle fibre is enclosed by a thin membrane containing many tiny fibres called myofibrils, which contain the active contractile elements. These are proteins called actin and myosin. In the contracted muscle the actin filaments and myosin filaments slide into each other to shorten the muscle length.

One fibre does not necessarily run the whole length of the muscle; rather, groups of fibres are connected to allow the force of contraction to be transmitted to the tendons. A muscle fibre has a length from 1–40 mm and a thickness from 0.01–1.10 mm. The muscle fibres are surrounded by a fine connective tissue with tiny blood vessels and nerves. A group of muscle fibres (a fasciculus) is surrounded by a connective tissue sheath, the perimysium.

Groups of muscle fibres are bound together to form the muscle, at the ends of which the connective tissue sheaths combine to become the tendons, which are fixed to a bone or other structure. Sometimes the attachment to the bone is via a large flat tendinous tissue called an aponeurosis. Some tendons are surrounded by a synovial sheath which is double-walled, containing a thin layer of synovial tissue on the inside and a layer of fibrous tissue on the sheath. Contraction of the muscle brings about movement at the joints.

Lying between and connected to the muscle fibres are muscle spindles, which are sensory receptors able to detect stretching of the muscle. They are deformed by stretching, and this provokes a motor response to contract the muscle fibres and shorten the muscle.

Muscle actions

- Muscles may contract or lengthen. They cannot on their own actively stretch or increase their length. However, a muscle may be actively lengthened by an outside force (gravity, for example). The muscle is then said to be working eccentrically. An example of this the action of the large front of thigh muscle, the quadriceps femoris, during the descent of the plié. The same muscle is said to be working concentrically during the ascent, when it is actively contracting against gravity and shortening.

- Muscles work in partnership with other muscles. As the quadriceps, for example, contracts to extend the knee, it acts as an agonist. At the same time, the opposite muscle group, the hamstrings, have to lengthen, and act as antagonists.

- A muscle which chiefly directs the action of a joint is called a prime mover. It initiates and produces the movement. Muscles which enable that movement to occur with the greatest efficiency are called fixators or stabilisers. Other muscles allow the body to isolate the action (that is, to keep other joints in a favourable position), and are called the synergists. All of these terms are relative to the action that is being performed.

The stretch reflex

It is important for the dance teacher to understand the stretch reflex. When a sudden stretch is placed on a muscle, a stretch receptor prevents damage to the muscle by bringing about a contraction of the muscle. These special receptors prevent the overstretching of a muscle by eliciting an automatic contraction of the muscle fibres; a reflex action. The amount and speed of the stretch is sensed by the muscle spindles. For dance teachers, particularly modern dance and jazz teachers, this information is important, as placing a sudden stretch on a muscle, as in a bounce forwards to stretch the hamstrings at the back of the thigh, will encourage that muscle to contract rather than producing the desired effect of stretching.

In order to stretch a muscle the stretch reflex must be not be provoked. This can be done by placing a slow, gradual stretch on a muscle. Opinions differ on how long the stretch needs to be held to overcome the reflex action, but it is generally held to be from one to several minutes.

*   *   *

Bones meet other bones to form joints. Those joints are moved and controlled by the action of muscles, which provide the force for the movement. Muscles, however, need to receive information on how much and when to contract. The nervous system provides this information by acting as a relay station between the thought and the action.

The nervous system

The nervous system is complex, so explanations will be as simple as possible, and therefore necessarily incomplete. (For further information see bibliography.)

The nervous system consists of the central nervous system, the peripheral nervous system and the autonomic nervous system. The central nervous system consists of the brain and the spinal cord. The peripheral nervous system sends and receives information from the limbs and extremities of the body to the spinal cord. It includes nerves which can send activity (motor) messages and receive information from the senses (sensory messages). The autonomic nervous system controls the digestion, lymphatic system and other systems inside the body.

The brain is a complex organ. The important centres for activity are the areas of the brain surface with special nerve cells. These nerve cells have nerve fibres going down into the spinal cord and from there into motor nerves of the body.

There are two types of nerve cells in the peripheral nervous system: the motor (or efferent) nerves, and the sensory (or afferent) nerves. The motor nerves initiate a reaction in a muscle and the sensory nerves sense the effect of that action and send feedback to the brain. The motor nerves arise from special cells called anterior horn cells in the spinal cord; the sensory nerves pass into the spinal cord from special cells called posterior horn cells.

Sensory nerves

In the skin, joints, muscles and tendons, and in many other places, there are special receptive organs giving information which is collected by sensory nerve endings, which in turn send messages back to the spinal cord. The sensory nerve fibres may end at the spinal cord, or go upwards to the brain. The fibres start with many fine nerve endings surrounded by a sensory nerve sheath of variable thickness. This thickness affects the quality of the sensations of touch, pressure, pain and temperature. From the joints and tendons come special sensory organs called the Golgi tendon organs. These are situated at the end of a muscle, just where it joins the tendon. Impulses from here give the brain information on tension in muscles.

Pressure on a sensory nerve can produce a feeling of numbness, or a 'pins and needles' sensation, or pain in the region from which the nerve fibres emanate. A mild degree of pressure on a nerve may cause a defect in the nerve function for some weeks. This is called neuropraxia. After regeneration of the nerve sheath the function should return to normal. With more severe compression of the nerve the sheath may be so damaged as to result in a defective nerve function.

Motor Nerves

To send a message to a muscle the brain sends an impulse down the spinal cord along the anterior horn cells. This is then transmitted to the nerve fibrils within a specific muscle by the signal crossing the neuromuscular junction in the muscle nerve cells. When the motor nerve reaches the muscle it splits into single nerve fibrils, each of which goes to the outside of a muscle fibre. A single nerve cell may innervate a number of muscle fibres. (If a single nerve cell is damaged or destroyed, all the muscle fibres in that group innervation will lose their function and die.) Muscle fibres belonging to a unit function simultaneously, the force of contraction depending on the number of activated motor nerves (the so-called 'recruitment' of muscle fibres). For a long-lasting muscle contraction, groups of muscle fibres will contract alternately.

Special systems

- *Muscle tone.* Muscle tone can be defined as the number of muscle fibres maintaining contraction in a muscle at rest. Tone is neurologically controlled and induced, and varies greatly from person to person. When a group of muscles is required to do a repetitive task such as maintaining the body in an upright position, it is less tiring for the body to do this by the muscle tone system than by conscious contraction of muscles. The ability of the body to assign repetitive movements to muscle tone is used fully by the dancer. In order to produce a movement over a long period of time, fibres can alternate recruitment to prevent fatigue. The brain decides how many fibres

24

need to be contracted to perform the movement. Muscle tone exists even in sleep; it is like a machine always ready for action.

Muscle tone is affected by many factors: emotional state (in a nervous or tense state more fibres are activated), general fitness, training, and temperature of the body. Excessive muscle tone maintains many muscle fibres in a state of contraction, which inhibits the extensibility of the muscles. This is called hypertonicity. Conversely, 'flabby' muscles have few fibres contracting at any one time; this is called hypotonicity. Neither extreme is very helpful for the dancer.

- *Proprioception.* Proprioception is a very special sense that tells the brain where the body is in space and where the limbs are in relationship to each other. It could be called a muscle, joint and tendon sense. The proprioceptors give sensory information to the brain. They detect motion and changes in the body even when the eyes are closed. Proprioception is an accumulation of several sensory receptors including information on tension (from the Golgi tendon organs) and length of muscles (from the muscle spindles). It is not fully understood how the brain processes all this information. The dancer uses these senses very acutely. Once a pattern of movement is learned – an arabesque, for example – the experienced body knows where to place the limbs and when the movement is 'in line', without looking in the mirror. Kinaesthetic awareness, a combination of feedback from proprioceptors and other sensory receptors, is very important for dancers.

*   *   *

Bones form joints, which are moved by muscles, which are in turn controlled by the nervous system. Sophisticated systems can tell the dancer where the body is and how it is performing. However, the special demands of dance training dictate that a more detailed knowledge of the structure of the dancer's body is necessary.

Part 2

The Structures

The vertebral column

The vertebral column consists of 33 irregular shaped bones called vertebrae. These bones are formed into four distinct curves of the spine and provide a wide range of movement. There are 7 vertebrae in the cervical spine (a secondary curve), 12 vertebrae in the thoracic spine (a primary curve), 5 vertebrae in the lumbar spine (a secondary curve), and 5 sacral bones in the sacrum (a primary curve). The last 3 or 4 vertebrae form the coccyx, and are fused together in adult life (Fig. 5).

The vertebrae have some common features. Each vertebra (except the first) has a solid body which consists of cancellous bone. In the back of the vertebra is a bony arch surrounding a hole – the vertebral foramen – for the spinal cord to pass through. On each side of the arch is a bony process called the transverse process. A further bony process projects backwards and is called the spinous process. These may be felt under the skin and are visible in thin individuals.

Between the bodies of adjacent vertebrae are found flat discs of fibro-cartilaginous tissue called the intervertebral discs. The centre of the disc has a jelly-like substance called the nucleus pulposus, which is surrounded by a tough outer fibrous layer called the annulus fibrosus. The discs can act as shock absorbers for the spine, and provide fluid movement while maintaining a connection from one vertebra to another. The gelatinous nature of the nucleus pulposus in the centre of the disc allows absorption of pressure as the spine moves by adapting to the shape of the spine. For example, if the dancer flexes laterally to the right, the disc will be compressed on the right side and not on the left side. The intervertebral discs increase in size in the cervical and lumbar spines, and are thicker anteriorly, thus contributing to the shape of the curves.

Between the laminae (plates of bone at the back of each vertebrae) are flat elastic yellow ligaments, connecting the spine. The joints between the articulating processes are synovial and have a joint capsule – like other joints – with the same disposition to painful diseases such as arthritis and osteoarthritis.

The cervical spine

There are 7 cervical vertebrae. The first, the atlas (C1), has a joint with the cranium – the atlanto-occipital joint. It is an atypical vertebra, as it has the

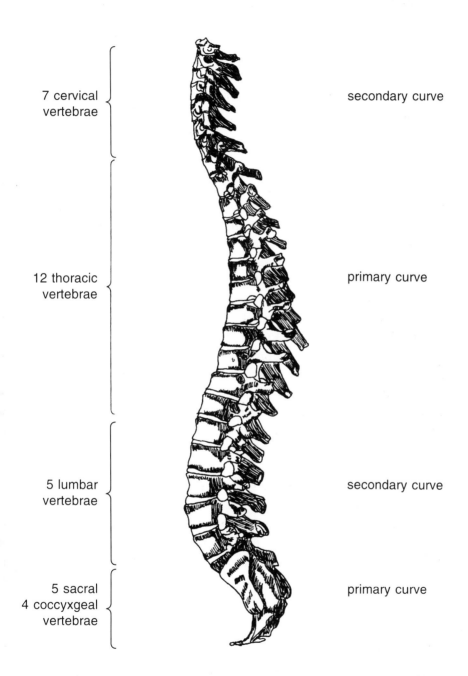

7 cervical
vertebrae

12 thoracic
vertebrae

5 lumbar
vertebrae

5 sacral
4 coccyxgeal
vertebrae

secondary curve

primary curve

secondary curve

primary curve

Fig. 5. The spine viewed from the left side, showing normal spinal curves.

form of a ring. The second cervical vertebra, the axis (C2), is also atypical as it has a special process like a peg projecting upwards into the front part of the atlas ring. This is called the odontoid process. The joint surfaces between the atlas and the axis (atlanto-axial joint) permit rotational movement, especially important in pirouettes. The range of movement in the cervical curve is flexion, extension, lateral flexion and rotation. It is the most mobile part of the spine.

The thoracic spine

The next part of the vertebral column is the thoracic curve, with 12 vertebrae. Connected to the side of these vertebrae are the ribs, each connected to the spine by the vertebral body and the transverse process. The joint with the body of the vertebra is called the costo-vertebral joint; the joint with the transverse process is called the costo-transverse joint. Anteriorly the ribs become cartilaginous. The cartilaginous part of the upper 10 ribs is connected to the flat breast bone, the sternum. The first 7 ribs are directly connected with the sternum, the next three are attached via costal cartilage to the rib above. The two lowest pairs of ribs are not connected to the sternum; they are the so-called 'floating ribs', although they do articulate with the transverse processes of the spine. The spinous processes of the thoracic vertebrae project down-wards and overlap each other, restricting movement backwards. Move-ment is generally limited in this curve because of the articulation with the rib cage, although rotation is possible with very little flexion and extension (Fig. 6).

The lumbar spine

The lowest part of the vertebral column, the lumbar curve, consists of 5 big vertebrae. The lowest (L5) is fixed to the upper surface of the sacral bone between the two hip bones at the back of the pelvic ring. The bodies of the lumbar vertebrae are massive, to support the increasing load of skeletal weight on the lower vertebrae. The spinous processes project directly backwards, and thus do not restrict any bending back-wards of the spine. The lumbar curve has a large range of movement, especially flexion and extension, but little rotation.

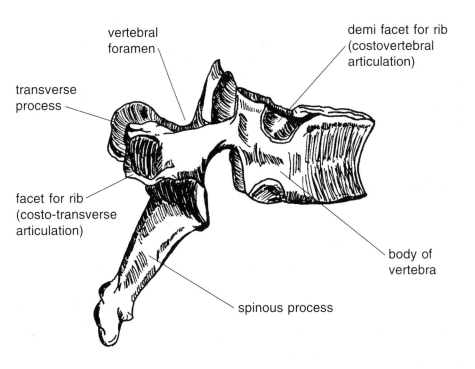

vertebral foramen

transverse process

demi facet for rib (costovertebral articulation)

facet for rib (costo-transverse articulation)

body of vertebra

spinous process

Fig. 6. A thoracic vertebra, viewed from the right side.

Sacral and coccyxgeal spine

The sacrum forms the posterior wall of the pelvis. The 5 sacral vertebrae are fused in adult life, and articulate laterally with the hip bone. This joint is called the sacro-iliac joint. It is an atypical synovial joint and allows only a small range of movement. This joint is subject to great strain, as it is where the weight of the body is transmitted diagonally downwards and sideways to the hip socket, the acetabulum. The sacro-iliac joint is reinforced with many supportive ligaments, but these may be subject to strain and be overstretched by forceful movements.

The remaining 3 or 4 vertebrae, the coccyxgeal bones, are also fused in adult life.

The vertebral foramina in each vertebra form a vertebral canal from the cranium downwards to the sacral bone. This canal contains the spinal cord from the brain down to the second lumbar vertebra (L2) and from this point a bundle of nerve fibres emerge called the cauda equina (so called because it looks like a horse's tail). Nerve fibres from the spinal cord and the cauda equina pass out through the vertebral canal through holes, the intervertebral foramina, formed between the roots of the vertebral arches.

Spinal abnormalities

- *Scoliosis.* Viewed from the back, the vertebral column should be straight, and any lateral curve is abnormal. Such a curve is called a scoliosis and the spine appears 'S'-shaped. If one leg is shorter than the other, when viewed from a standing position, the pelvis and the sacral bones will be tilted and the spine will show a lateral curvature. The lowest part of the vertebral column will be curved to the side of the shorter leg. In sitting and in standing position with the body bent forwards, this scoliosis may disappear. If a dancer has a such a scoliosis, the shorter leg may be compensated for by elevating the leg with a heel cushion in the shoe. (The length of the legs can be evaluated from the back with one hand on the upper part of each hip bone.)

  A serious type of scoliosis is caused by a deformity of the vertebrae. The vertebral bodies have a 'wedge' shape and one side of the vertebral column has a convex curvature towards the side where the body of the vertebrae is highest. There is often a rotation of the vertebrae in the scoliotic part of the column. The bodies of the vertebrae are turned to the convex side, and the result of this torsion is a prominence on the back of the ribs, by the transverse processes on the convex side of the scoliosis. This torsion prominence is typical of an organic scoliosis and it is most easily seen in the middle of the spine when the dancer bends the body forwards.

  Some cases of scoliosis develop during the growth period with little indication as to the cause. This is called idiopathic scoliosis. The most common location of the scoliotic curve is in the thoracic column, and there will always be corresponding curves to the opposite direction above and below the primary position of the scoliosis. Idiopathic scoliosis is most common in girls with a right thoracic primary curve. It tends to appear at the age of 9–11, and the severity of the curve may increase until growth has stopped at the age of 14–16.

  Any marked degree of scoliosis must be examined and controlled by an orthopaedic surgeon. The extent of the scoliotic curve is measured as the degree of the angle between the lines of the first and last vertebrae as seen on an X-ray in the standing position. A scoliosis with a primary curve up to 15–20 degrees does not need treatment but should be monitored with X-rays taken during the growth period. If the degree of scoliosis is higher than 20 degrees, treatment must be considered, and the student should be advised to discontinue dance training.

A mild degree of postural scoliosis may be seen in adolescents. This may be caused by postural bad habits, or the overuse of one side of the spine, such as by always carrying a heavy school bag on the same shoulder. The relaxed, non-dance standing position should be examined and checked for correct alignment of the spine. Postural scoliosis can usually be corrected by changing the habit that caused it.

- *Kyphosis.* The normal curve of the thoracic spine is a slight backwards convex curve. An exaggerated kyphosis with wedge-shaped vertebral bodies causes a round back. If this develops during the growing years of adolescence it is called Scheuermann's kyphosis. This is often accompanied by an exaggerated lumbar curve. A spine of this type is not suitable for dance training.
- *Lordosis.* Lordosis is the term given to the normal forwards (concave) curve in the lumbar spine. Confusingly, it is also the name given to the abnormality of an exaggerated curve. Causes of increased lordosis may be postural bad habits (often with corresponding weak abdominal muscles), or a congenital abnormality. If the curve is very exaggerated the spine will be too weak to cope with the demands of classical training. Young children usually appear to have lordosis until the 'baby' tummy has disappeared and strong abdominal muscles are able to control the pelvis.

If the exaggerated lordosis is congenital, the spine is unlikely to be suitable for full-time vocational training, although recreational dance classes will probably help correct some weaknesses.

Posture

The normal curves of the spine are decreased by the technical demands of ballet (Plates 1 & 2). The 'flat' back is seen as aesthetically desirable. This, however, decreases the ability of the spine to act as a shock-

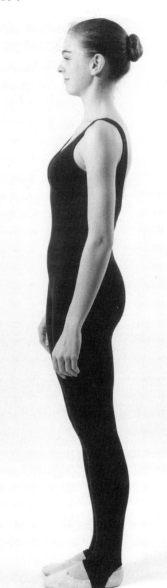

Plate 1. The natural curves of the spine with the dancer in a relaxed position.

absorber, and the flattening of the normal curves can have adverse effects. An adult dancer with a 'flat' back has a tendency to lower back pain caused by degeneration of the lower intervertebral discs. Sometimes a reversal of the normal curves is seen with a lordosis in the thoracic curve and a kyphotic lumbar curve.

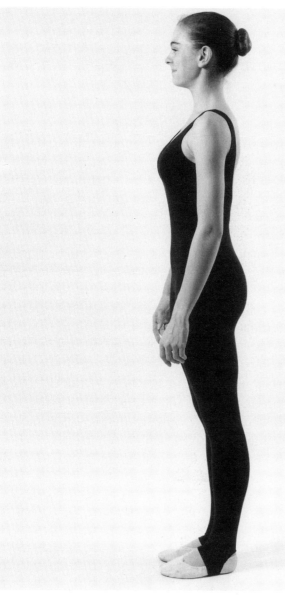

Plate 2. The lengthened position with decreased curves of the spine and central line of gravity place on the middle of the foot.

A fast-growing child with weak muscles may exhibit poor posture with correctable kyphosis, lordosis and prominent tummy and shoulder blades. With training and time these usually disappear as muscles mature.

For the dancer the ideal posture is to have the centre of the body in a line from above the ears, to the centre of the shoulders, centre of the pelvis, centre of the knee, through the ankle to the centre of the foot.

Muscles which move the spine

Cervical curve

Muscles attached to the occipital bone of the cranium balance the head on top of the spinal column.

- At the side of the head is the long sternocleidomastoid muscle, which has an origin behind the ear and inserts into the medial end of the clavicle (collar bone). This and other muscles at the front of the head move the head in different directions and rotate the head.
- The trapezius muscle has its origin in the cervical vertebrae and is responsible for some actions of the head and neck.

Sensory and motor nerves come through the intervertebral foramina at the cervical curve and go to the arm.

Thoracic curve

- The trapezius, which has its origins at the base of the skull, runs down to the twelfth thoracic vertebra, and inserts into the scapula and clavicle. It acts on the shoulder by moving the scapula upwards, downwards and rotating the scapula.
- The erector spinae is a long, thick muscle running the length of the vertebrae at the sides of the spinous processes.
- The latissimus dorsi is a large muscle that originates along the borders of the spinous processes from T7 down to the posterior surface of the ilium. It inserts into the medial aspect of the humerus, and acts to draw the arm downwards and to rotate it inwards. It is a very important muscle for men when partnering, as it aids in controlling the lowering of the female dancer from an overhead position.
- Other muscles which act upon the thoracic curve are discussed on pages 43–44.

Nerves emanate from the spinal cord through holes at the side of the thoracic column. They are then located in the muscles between the muscles of the ribs and abdominal muscles.

Lumbar curve

The lumbar curve is flexed by the abdominal muscles at the front of the body. These are:

- The rectus abdominis, which runs up the front of the abdomen from the pubic symphysis to the ribs. It flexes the trunk and is responsible for helping the dancer to sit up from a lying down position.
- The external oblique, which runs in a diagonal across the trunk. The internal oblique runs diagonally opposite to the external oblique. Their combined actions rotate the trunk, twisting it to one side.
- The transversus abdominis, as its name suggests, runs across the front of the abdomen. It pulls the stomach in.

Other muscles of the lower back:

- The psoas is a long muscle originating in the front of the lumbar vertebral bodies, and runs downwards and forwards. At the anterior of the pelvis it joins another muscle, the iliacus, and continues to run forwards over the pubic bone to insert at the end of the femoral neck. Here it is called the iliopsoas. This important muscle flexes the hip joint and bends the lumbar column forwards.
- The quadratus lumborum runs from the lower ribs to the posterior part of the iliac crest. It can act to produce lateral flexion of the spine and also extension of the spine.

Most of the nerves that exit from the lumbar curve form what is called a plexus, a network of nerves and blood vessels. The first part of the lumbar plexus is located in the psoas muscle; it then runs downwards to form the big femoral nerve at the front of the thigh.

The nerve network from the lower lumbar curve and the sacral curve exits from the vertebral foramina and the holes in the sacral bones, forming the sacral plexus. This is a large network of peripheral nerves from the hip region, and includes the sciatic nerve, which runs down the thigh and leg to end in the tibial and peroneal nerves.

Possible spinal problems

- If an intervertebral disc is subject to damage or degeneration, the outer annulus fibrosus of the disc may rupture and allow the inner gelatinous material to bulge backwards, putting pressure onto the spinal cord and the nerves passing behind the disc (commonly called a 'slipped disc'). This will cause pain which passes into the legs. A symptom of such nerve pressure would be an inability to do a straight leg raise. Another possible case of nerve damage may be from the first sacral nerve on the lowest lumbar disc, which would result in a impairment of the Achilles tendon reflex.

- Injury or pressure on the fifth lumbar nerve and the first sacral nerve often manifests itself as atrophy and reduced power in the leg, the hip muscles, and the lower leg muscles, especially the toe extensors (which flex the foot upwards). This is the effect of damage to the motor nerves.
- Any sensory nerve damage at the L5–S1 junction will be manifested in the foot. The dorsum (upper surface) of the foot and the lateral (outside) surface of the foot will have reduced sensation. Damage to this area may be seen on an X-ray as a narrowing of the joint space between two vertebra and a corresponding narrowing of the intervertebral disc. A whole body scan will also demonstrate the disc protrusion.
- Stress fractures of the vertebrae are unfortunately common in dancers, particularly male dancers. This is often due to frequent weight loading on the spine when lifting partners. A stress fracture is a response to repeated excessive stress in an bone.

* * *

The spine provides the upright framework for the body. The lower limbs are directly connected to the spine by the pelvis. The upper limbs are not directly connected to the spine at all, but the shoulder blade glides over the upper back to give a special range of movement.

The shoulder and arm

The bones of the arm are:
- The clavicle (collar bone) which joins the arm to the body
- The scapula (or shoulder blade)
- The humerus (the long upper arm bone)
- The radius and the ulna (the lower arm bones)
- The 8 carpal bones (wrist bones)
- The 5 metacarpal bones (middle hand bones)
- The phalanges (the fingers and thumb)

Structure

Shoulder

The shoulder is a synovial ball-and-socket joint. Its correct anatomical name is the glenohumeral joint.

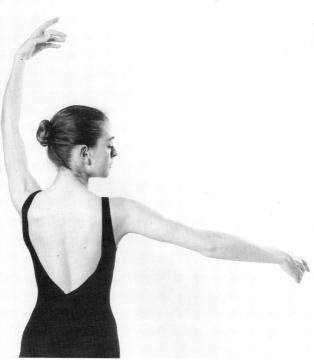

Plate 3. The shoulder and arms.

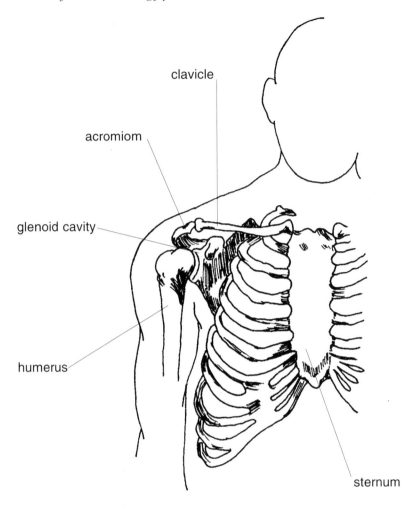

Fig. 7. The right shoulder joint viewed from the front.

- At the lateral apex of the flat triangular scapula (shoulder blade) is an oval socket called the glenoid cavity. The round head of the upper arm bone, the humerus, articulates with the glenoid cavity to form the shoulder joint. The range of movement permitted here is quite free: flexion, extension, adduction, abduction, rotation and a combination of circular movements called circumduction. The scapula, held in place only by strong muscles, slides around the thorax to facilitate

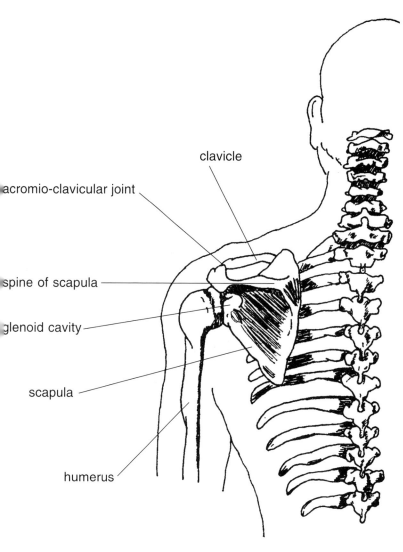

clavicle

acromio-clavicular joint

spine of scapula

glenoid cavity

scapula

humerus

Fig. 8. The left shoulder joint viewed from the back.

movement. Movements at the shoulder are a combination of gleno-humeral movement and scapula motion (Fig. 7).
• On the back of the scapula is a bony ridge called the spine of the scapula. This ends in a bony crest at the height of the shoulder called the acromiom. This can be easily felt under the skin. The acromiom

then connects with the clavicle (collar bone) at the distal end of the shoulder in a joint called the acromioclavicular joint. It is stabilised by a ligament on the undersurface of the clavicle, permitting very little movement. Dislocation after a fall on this joint is very common, as there is little joint protection at the front (Fig. 8).

- The clavicle is connected medially to the sternum (breast bone) at a joint called the sternoclavicular joint. The joint is stabilised by a very strong ligament between the clavicle and the first rib; therefore a dislocation at this joint is very rare. The sternoclavicular joint is the only fixed attachment of the shoulder (and hence of the arm) to the body.

- The shoulder joint has a lax capsule which allows a great range of movement. The tendons of the muscles at the front and back of the scapula are interwoven with the muscles around the shoulder joint. This is collectively called the rotator cuff, and runs around the edge of the socket to bony projections of the humerus. The muscles that comprise the rotator cuff are the infraspinatus, teres minor, supraspinatus and subscapularis. They help to stabilise the glenohumeral joint and hold the humerus in the shallow glenoid cavity.

- The shoulder and scapula are involved in the movement of the arm. The humerus is set into the glenoid cavity at an approximately 30-degree angle forwards. The arm may be raised to first and second position with little movement in the scapula, but as the arm moves above the head to fifth position or to arabesque positions, the scapula moves around the thorax to permit the movement.

- The humerus is a long bone with the upper end forming the round ball to fit into the socket of the shoulder. At the superior (upper) end there are two bony projections called tubercles for muscle attachments. The distal (lower) end by the elbow is flatter and broader with two prominent processes which articulate with the lower arm bones.

Elbow

The radius and the ulna articulate with the humerus, forming the elbow joint. At the lower end of the humerus is a fossa (a hollow depression called the olecranon fossa, which meets a reciprocally shaped extension of the ulna, called the olecranon. This is the sharp corner of the elbow which prevents overextension of the joint. The elbow joint is primarily a hinge joint with stabilising ligaments on the sides. The front and back of the joint has a lax capsule which allows free movement.

It is possible to move the lower arm inwards and outwards (pronation and supination) with the humerus fixed. The dancer uses this slight rotational movement when holding the arm in second position. The upper arm is held in a slight inwards rotation, the lower arm in a slightly supinated position. This rotational movement in the elbow is facilitated by the spherical head of the radius meeting a concave surface on the small epicondyle of the humerus, and a similar small head of the ulna meeting a concave surface on the lower end of the radius. There is a fibrous disc on the radius which connects with a small process on the ulna (the styloid process) which binds the two bones together.

Wrist
The wrist joint is formed by the surfaces of the radius and the ulna articulating with the carpal bones. This joint may be moved forwards and backwards to about 60–70 degrees, about 10 degrees inwards towards the thumb, and about 30 degrees outwards towards the fifth finger. The combined movements of the fingers and thumb provide a wide range of movements for the hand.

Muscles affecting the arm

- The latissimus dorsi originates by the ilium, spinous processes of the lumbar vertebrae and the last three ribs. It then moves diagonally upwards to insert into the upper humerus. One of the actions of the latissimus dorsi can be best felt by the dancer when controlling the descent of the arm from second position to bras bas. It also acts to move the arm backwards, as in arabesque épaulement.
- The large triangular trapezius muscle originates in the skull and along the spinous processes of the cervical and thoracic vertebrae. It then inserts into the spine of the scapula, out to the acromiom process and the lateral edge of the clavicle. This muscle lifts the whole arm and rotates the scapula.
- The serratus anterior muscle covers the lateral part of the thorax underneath the scapula. This pulls the scapula, and therefore the arm, forwards.

- At the anterior part of the thorax is the large pectoralis major muscle. This muscle pulls the arm forwards and rotates it inwards.
- On the lateral side of the shoulder is the deltoid muscle, which gives the rounded shape to the shoulder. The deltoid comes from the acromiom, the clavicle and the spine of the scapula and inserts to the shaft of the humerus. It moves the upper arm outwards (for example, when lifting the arm to second position from bras bas).
- On the upper arm are the long muscles for flexion and extension of the elbow. The biceps are in front of the arm, and the antagonists, the triceps, on the back of the arm.
- In the lower arm there are many muscles for flexion and extension, pronation and supination of the wrist, and many muscles to move the fingers.
- The hands have many small muscles to move the fingers and produce the fine, delicate movements that a dancer needs. Female dancers need to have very expressive arms and male dancers need very strong arms and handgrips to support the female in pas de deux. The male dancer must have strong shoulders and arms to enable him to lift his partner in the air.

*   *   *

In many ways the shoulder joint and the hip joint are very similar. However, the shoulder is not a weight-bearing joint (apart from when male dancers lift female dancers on to their shoulders!) and as such has a wider range of movement than the hip joint, which has to take the axial weight of the body.

The hip and thigh

The bones of the hip are:

- The os innominatum: ilium
                    ischium } form acetabulum or socket
                    pubis
- The femur

The hip bone, or os innominatum, is in fact three bones. The large, wing-shaped upper part is called the ilium. The ischium and the pubis form the lower third of the hip bone. All three bones unite in the hip socket, which is called the acetabulum. The hip joint is found on the lateral aspect of the pelvis, which can be thought of as a bony ring made up of the two hip bones and the sacrum. Posteriorly, the hip bones form a joint with the upper part of the sacrum (the large bony triangle at the base of the spine) called the sacroiliac joint. Anteriorly, the two pubic bones meet each other to form the pubic symphysis. The pubic bone is then directed backwards and downwards to become the ischium, ending in a thickened prominence called the ischial tuberosity. We know these more commonly as the 'sitting bones'. The three bones of the acetabulum do not fuse together until adult life. During childhood there is cartilage radiating between the bones in the acetabulum.

Structure

- The hip joint is a ball-and-socket joint with a wide range of movement: flexion and extension; medial rotation and lateral rotation; abduction and adduction; and a combination of these movements called circumduction. The joint capsule is very strong around the joint except at the back. At the front is a thick ligament called the iliofemoral ligament (or Y-shaped ligament) which runs from the upper rim of the acetabulum to the base of the neck of the femur and the lesser trochanter of the femur. The ligament has a horizontal and a vertical part. Two other important ligaments around the hip joint are the pubofemoral and the ischiofemoral ligaments. These run around the neck of the femur and prevent backwards extension of the hip. Inside the fibrous capsule is the synovial capsule which secretes synovial

45

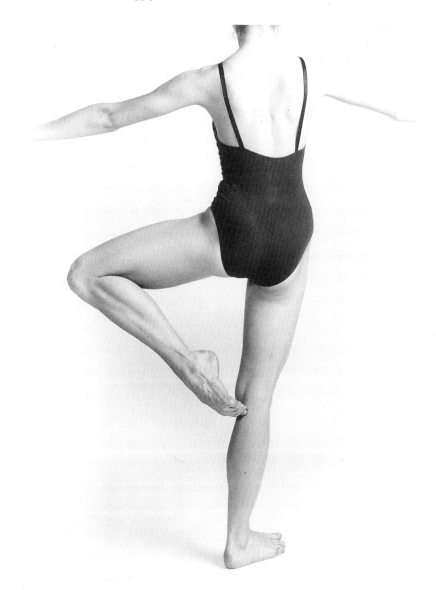

Plate 4. The hip joint.

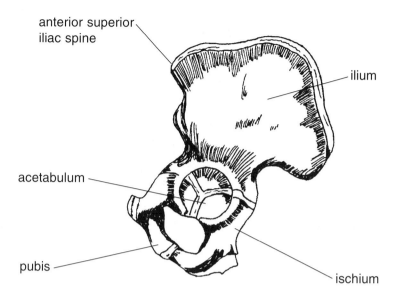

anterior superior iliac spine

ilium

acetabulum

pubis

ischium

Fig. 9. The left hip bone viewed from the side.

fluid to lubricate the joint. In children and adolescents the epiphyseal scar is at the base of the head of the femur (Fig. 9).

- The iliac bone, with a large bony spine at the anterior superior edge, can be seen and felt in slim people. It is called the anterior superior iliac spine. From the outside of the ilium important gluteal muscles originate, including the gluteus maximus, which inserts to the greater trochanter of the femur.
- The acetabulum of the hip joint is on the lateral side of the hip bone. It is angled about 35 degrees forwards and 15 degrees downwards. The acetabulum is semi-spherical in shape. At the back of the acetabulum, above the ischium, is a foramen (the greater sciatic foramen) for the passage of nerves from the sacral plexus.
- The femur is the longest bone in the body. The upper end has a semi-spherical head which is covered in articular cartilage. From the head of the femur there is a strong ligament called the ligamentum teres which attaches the femur into the acetabulum (Fig. 10). The neck of

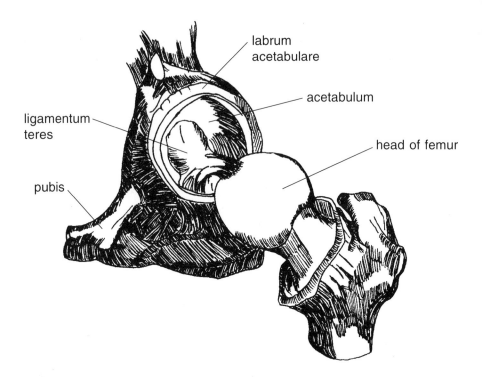

Fig. 10. The left hip socket, with head of femur displaced from the acetabulum to show the ligamentum teres.

the femur directs the weight diagonally sideways and forwards, and ends with two prominences called the greater and lesser trochanters. The angle between the femoral shaft and the neck is normally about 120 degrees. The lower part of the femur ends in two large 'knuckles', called condyles, which articulate at the knee with the shin bone.

Factors governing turn-out

- The depth of the acetabulum. The deeper the socket, the less turn-out will be facilitated. The actual shape of the socket is also a predetermining factor.
- The angle of the neck of the femur. At the upper end of the femur, the neck of the femur inclines inwards towards the socket. This angulation is important for a dancer's turn-out.

- The length of the neck of the femur.
- The elasticity of the iliofemoral ligament. Also known as the Y-shaped ligament, this is situated at the front of the hip joint and shaped like an inverted 'Y'. It is a very strong ligament.
- The age at which dance training began. The sooner the iliofemoral ligament is encouraged to stretch and facilitate movement, the more turn-out a dancer is likely to have.

Of all the above factors, only the last one can affect a change in turn-out. All the other factors are predetermined congenital factors. However, it is possible to strengthen the muscles that control the turn-out in order to maximise full facility.

Examining the mobility of the hip joint

The mobility of the hip joint should be examined with the dancer lying down.

- Extend one leg up to its maximum position with the other hip (supporting side) still and extended. If there is a defect in the hip joint due to a contracture or osteoarthrosis, the extended hip will be moved into flexion. This is called the Thomas test.
- The amount of flexion in a joint is measured in degrees from the extended position (zero). Usually it is about 150 degrees. However, it is important to ascertain that pure hip movement is measured, as the spine and pelvis may be engaged in facilitating the flexion. Other factors such as muscle bulk may inhibit measurements.
- By moving an extended leg out to the side the abduction of the joint can be measured. Usually it is about 45 degrees.
- By moving the extended leg medially across the body, adduction can be measured. It is normally about 30 degrees.
- Rotation of the joint should be measured with the dancer lying prone (face down). The knee is bent up to about 90 degrees and the lower leg is then moved outwards to measure internal rotation and then inwards to measure the important external rotation (turn-out).

It is common for dance students to have unequal lateral rotation at the hip joint. This may cause problems if the dancer turns out both feet to the extent of the most turned-out leg.

Adolescent problems at the hip joint

There are three main problems associated with children in the hip joint.

- Legg-Perthes disease is a change of the shape of bone at the femoral head. Normal bone tissue dies from lack of blood supply and the epiphysis is partly dissolved. Later the structure regenerates growth but often with a flattening of the femoral head. Young dancers experiencing this problem will first notice pain in the area especially on movement of abduction (taking the leg away from the body). Pain may sometimes be referred to the knee, which can cause a delay in diagnosis. This problem is mostly found in young boys aged between 5 and 10 years.
- Another hip disease specific to children is epiphysiolysis of the femoral head. This is damage to the growth cartilage at the epiphyseal scar. Bone change here allows the head of the femur to dislocate downwards and backwards. Painful internal rotation is a characteristic symptom of this problem, although pain may be also experienced in the hip or knee area. This is most common in adolescent boys.
- Arthritis is an inflammation of the joint where all movements are painful. All activity should stop with this condition.

Muscles of the hip region

- The gluteus maximus is the largest muscle in the body. It forms the buttock muscle, and is especially visible in dancers. The muscle arises from the back of the sacrum and the outside of the ilium. It inserts in two ways: it is fixed to the back of the femur, and it also inserts into a large flat tendon on the outside of the thigh into the iliotibial band. The action of the gluteus maximus rotates the thigh laterally, and extends the hip. In the standing position it can change the tilt of the pelvis by working with the rectus abdominis at the front of the pelvis. This will bring the pelvis into an upright position by tilting the pelvis backwards. The gluteus maximus must be used as a turn-out muscle in conjunction with other turn-out muscles. There is a tendency amongst dancers to use this muscle excessively by holding too much tension in it.
- The other gluteus muscles are the minimus and the medius. The gluteus minimus is an important postural muscle, as it balances the body on the pelvis when the dancer stands on one leg. For the dancer

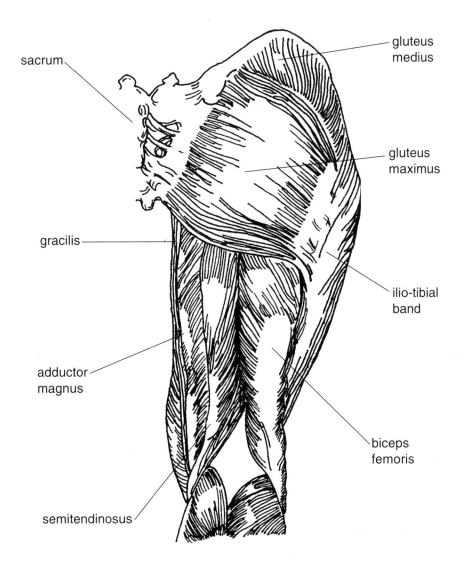

Fig. 11. The right posterior hip and thigh muscles.

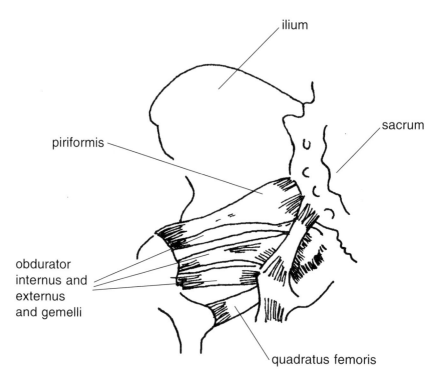

Fig. 12. The left posterior hip showing six deep lateral rotators, piriformis, obturators internus and externus, gemelli superior and inferior, and quadratus femoris.

this action is very important when the dancer needs a strong supporting side. Insufficient strength in this muscle will cause the dancer to appear to 'sit into' the hip. The actions of the gluteus medius also aid in balancing the body on one leg, and it is commonly believed that it acts as a medial rotator of the femur (Fig. 11).

- A smaller flatter muscle in the hip region is the tensor fascia latae. This arises from the front part of the iliac crest and inserts below the greater trochanter of the femur and into the iliotibial band. It also has the action of positioning the pelvis when standing on one leg.
- Six deep lateral rotator muscles are very important for the dancer. They cross the hip joint posteriorly, arising from the pelvis and inserting into the posterior aspect of the greater trochanter of the femur.

They are: the piriformis; the gemelli superior and inferior; the obturators internus and externus; and the quadratus femoris. Their combined actions aid lateral rotation (turn-out), and they also function during standing and walking (Fig. 12).

- The iliopsoas muscle arises from the lumbar vertebrae and the inside of the ilium, and inserts into the lesser trochanter of the femur. It is important for flexing the hip and for posture.
- On the inside of the thigh is the group of muscles known as the adductors. They are the adductors longus, brevis and magnus. They arise from the lower curve of the pubic and ischial bones and insert into the back of the femur. Their action is best thought of in the grand rond de jambe en dedans: adducting the hip while maintaining lateral rotation in a flexed hip position. When standing on one leg the adductors pull one leg towards the other. Encouraging dancers to imagine using these muscles will often promote good muscle action, but it is very difficult for the dancer to use these muscles in isolation from other accessory lateral rotators.
- At the back of the thigh are the hamstring muscles. These are the biceps femoris, semitendinosus and semimembranosus. They all arise from the ischial tuberosity (the sitting bones) and run down the back of the thigh. The biceps femoris inserts into the fibula on the outside of the leg. The semimembranosus ends with a big tendon on the back of the medial tibial condyle. The thinner semitendinosus runs with the gracilis (an adductor) and the sartorius (a hip flexor) to the inside of the knee by the upper part of the tibia, and inserts via a common tendon called the pes anserinus. The hamstrings flex the knee and extend the hip (lift the leg backwards). They are also responsible for bringing the body to an upright position after a forwards port de bras.
- At the front of the thigh is the large quadriceps femoris group. There are four muscles in this group: the rectus femoris, the vastus medialis, the vastus lateralis, and the vastus intermedius. The rectus femoris is the only one which acts over two joints (the hip and the knee), as it has its origin above the acetabulum. The four muscles form a common tendon in which the patella lies at the front of the knee. The insertion of the quadriceps is by a tendon into the tibial tuberosity. This tendon also has another name, the patellar ligament – which is confusing, as it is not a ligament (Fig. 13).

The action of the quadriceps is to flex the hip and extend the knee.

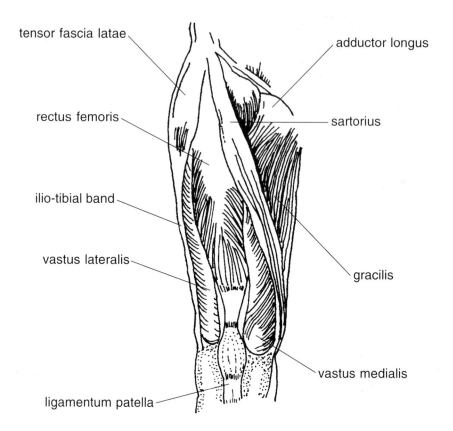

tensor fascia latae

adductor longus

rectus femoris

sartorius

ilio-tibial band

vastus lateralis

gracilis

vastus medialis

ligamentum patella

Fig. 13. The right thigh and knee joint showing quadriceps femoris and other anterior thigh muscles.

The vastus medialis is important for dancers as it is responsible for the last few degrees of extension of the knee, therefore it is important that it is strong to maintain the integrity of the close packed position of the joint when under stress from maintaining fifth position of the legs.

• The sartorius is the longest muscle in the body, and originates from the anterior superior iliac spine. It then runs diagonally downwards and across the front of the thigh (it is often visible in well trained dancers with good muscle tone) and inserts into the medial aspect of

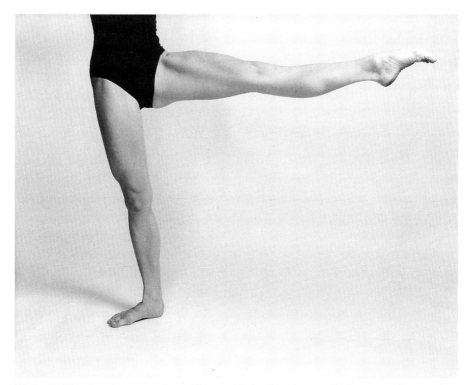

Plate 5. The leg in second position en l'air showing sartorius muscle running across the thigh.

the tibia. It aids in hip flexion, outward rotation (especially in attitude devant) and flexion of the knee. It is a two-joint muscle (Plate 5).

- The gracilis is often termed an adductor as it lies so close to the adductor group of muscles. It originates in the pubis and runs diagonally downwards to insert into the medial aspect of the tibia. It aids adduction of the hip, flexion of the knees, and internal rotation of the hip.

*   *   *

The hip joint transmits the weight of the body from the upright spine onto the two legs. The relationship with the knee joint is very intricate, especially for a dancer who uses the lateral rotator facility of the hips. Correct alignment of these two joints is critical for healthy knees.

The knee

The bones of the knee are:
- The femur
- The tibia
- The patella

The knee is a synovial condyloid hinge joint. It is an articulation between the femoral condyles and the tibia (shin bone). The smaller fibula bone on the lateral side of the tibia does not form part of the knee joint, but articulates only with the tibia. The knee capsule is very strong at the back and sides of the joint. The movement of the femoral condyles is rolling and gliding on the tibia. The range of movement available at the knee is flexion and extension, with some rotation allowed when the joint is flexed (for example when performing a rond de jambe en l'air).

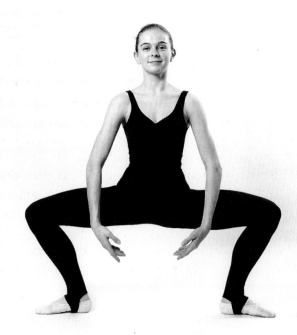

Plate 6. The knee joints in action.

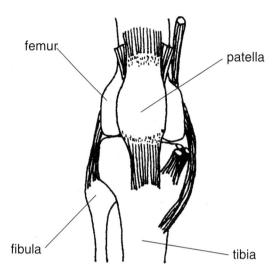

Fig. 14. The right thigh and knee joint viewed from the front.

- The large femoral condyles are convex and fit into the concave surfaces of the reciprocating tibial condyles. As the tibial condyles have
fairly shallow depressions, there are two menisci lining the semicircular surface of the tibia to deepen the shallow concavity. These
menisci (also known as semi-lunar cartilages) are of tough fibrocartilage and are crescent-shaped. There is a medial and lateral meniscus. They guide and control the movement of the femoral condyles on
the tibia and also to some extent act as shock-absorbers.
- The patella (knee cap) is a small sesamoid bone (a bone embedded in
a tendon). The tendon in this case is that of the large quadriceps
muscle at the front of the thigh. The patella acts as a lever for this
muscle to work through an angle when the knee is bent. The back of
the patella is grooved slightly to an apex for articulation with the large
femoral condyles. The patella articulates only with the femur (Fig. 14).

Stabilising structures of the knee

- At the sides of the knee are stabilising ligaments. These run down both sides of the knee and connect the femur with the fibula on the lateral side and with the tibia on the medial side. They are called the collateral ligaments. The medial collateral ligament runs from the condyle of the femur to the medial side of the tibia. It also has a link with the medial meniscus. The lateral collateral ligament runs from the outside of the condyle of the femur down to the head of the fibula.

- On the inside of the knee are two ligaments which cross over inside the joint. They are the cruciate ligaments, and form an 'X'-shape in the knee. The anterior cruciate ligament connects the front of the tibia to the back of the femur; the posterior cruciate ligament connects the back of the tibia to the front of the femur. These ligaments help stabilise the knee. In extension they rotate the femur inwards about 5 degrees. It is rare for a dancer to have problems with these ligaments, which are more commonly injured in contact sports such as football or rugby.

- At the front of the knee the tendon of the quadriceps femoris acts as a ligament to stabilise the joint. This tendon is often referred to as the patellar ligament, although it is in fact a tendon. It inserts into the small bump at the front of the tibia called the tibial tuberosity.

- The retinaculae are flat tendons that help keep the patella in place when the knee is flexed and extended.

- At the back of the knee are strong tendons to stabilise the knee. These are:
  - the tendon of the semimembranosus (a hamstring muscle), which runs down the back of the thigh to the medial condyle of the tibia.
  - the tendon of the biceps femoris (a hamstring muscle), which runs down the back of the thigh to the head of the fibula.
  - the iliotibial band (a strong tough tissue), running down the outside of the thigh to the lateral tibial condyle.
  - the tendons of the gastrocnemius (the large calf muscle), which support the stability of the extended knee.

The whole knee joint is encased in a joint capsule which in turn is lined with a synovial capsule. This arises from the edge of the joint surfaces and covers the fibrous joint capsule. There are folds of the synovia at the sides of the patella. If there is damage to the joint there will be an accumulation of synovial fluid in the joint and these folds will distend, with visible swelling of the knee.

Bursae around the knee

Around the knee are several bursae (little sacs of synovial fluid). They serve to aid in friction-free movement between two surfaces. If irritated they respond by swelling with more synovial fluid and cause pain and tenderness. There are many bursae around the knee. Most commonly injured are:

- The prepatellar bursa, at the front of the patella between the bone and the skin.
- The suprapatellar bursa, at the front of the knee between the front of the femur and the end of the quadriceps tendon.
- The infrapatellar subcutaneous bursa, at the front of the tibial tuberosity (the attachment of the tendon of the quadriceps).
- The deep infrapatellar bursa, at the back of this same insertion of the tendon on the tibial tuberosity.
- Several bursae at the back of the knee around the hamstring tendons.
- The pes anserinus bursa, also at the back of the knee by the combined insertions of the sartorius, gracilis and semitendinosus. This may be the site of some pain at the back of the knee and the bursa may be tender and painful.

Abnormalities of the knee

- *Knock knees* (genu valgum). This is when the angle of the femur brings the knees together when the legs are placed passively in parallel. Knock-kneed dancers often have accompanying rolling ankles, as the weight of the body is incorrectly transmitted through the inside of the leg. Dancers with this problem should be encouraged to support the legs in parallel with muscle action and should not be made to stand with the legs touching when in parallel. Dancers with knock knees do not have an appealing aesthetic line and any severe degree of abnormality is not suitable for professional training (Plates 7 & 8).
- *Bow legs* (genu varum). This is when the legs curve slightly outwards when placed in parallel. The weight of the body tends to be transmitted towards the lateral side of the leg. Bow legs are not as weak as knock knees but again any severe degree will hamper the accepted aesthetic line. Bow-legged dancers tend to have strong muscular legs and will often have a strong jump.
- *Swayback legs* (genu recurvatum or hyperextended knees). This is

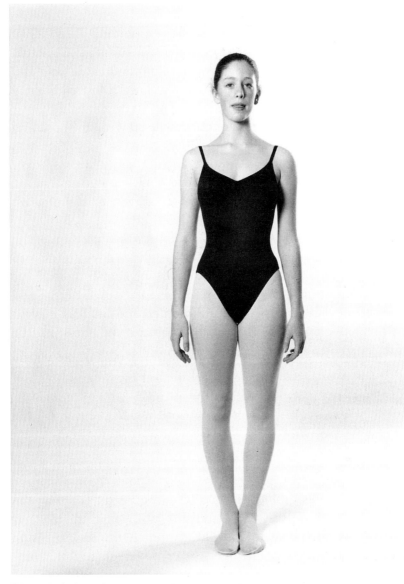

Plate 7. A 'bow leg' dancer in a relaxed position.

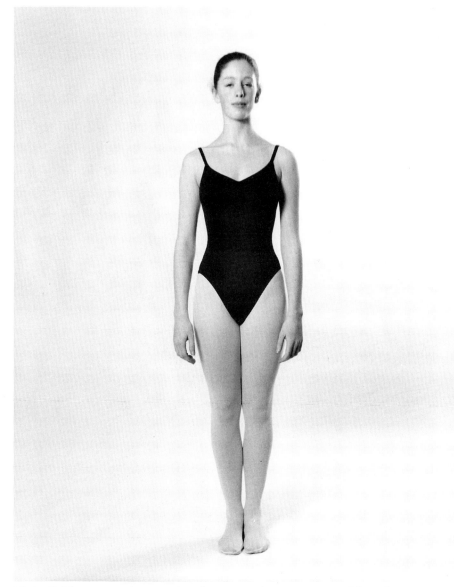

Plate 8. The same dancer showing muscular correction of bow legs.

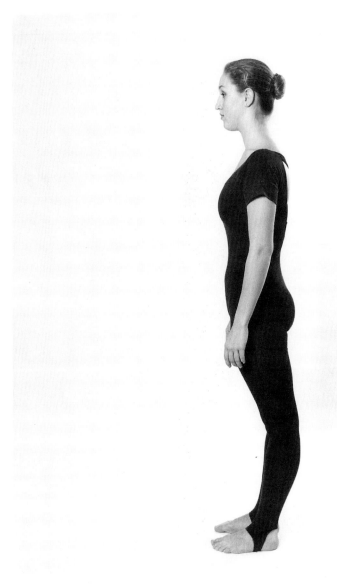

Plate 9. A 'swayback leg' dancer in a relaxed position.

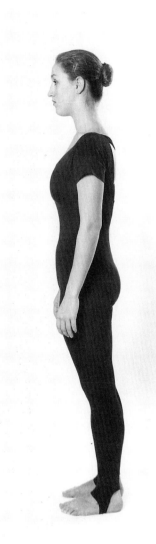

Plate 10. The same dancer showing muscular correction of swayback legs.

when the knees appear to curve backwards. This is commonly accepted as being the most aesthetically appealing shape of leg for a dancer. Unfortunately it is also a very unstable leg, with a high predisposition for injury. Dancers with swayback legs often have a chain reaction of musculo-skeletal problems: hyperlordosis and overarched feet. Swayback legs do not withstand jumps well, as the central line of gravity of the body is not correctly transmitted through the body. This is a particularly difficult shape of leg to train, as the leg must not be allowed to relax backwards into the hyperextended position. Strong muscles of the quadriceps and hamstrings will help support this shape of leg (Plates 9 & 10).

Common problems of the knee

The knee joint is a highly complex and intricate joint. Consequently, when injured it tends to be a serious problem. This is exacerbated by the fact that the quadriceps muscle atrophies very quickly, adding to the general instability of the joint. Many problems of the knee are caused by incorrect use.

- A common problem in the knee is pain on the medial aspect of the knee. This is often due to incorrect weight placement onto the inside of the knee joint (and may be related to poor turn-out from the hip on the injured side). This may lead to damage of the medial meniscus. Less common is damage of the lateral meniscus.

  Such lesions may be accompanied by a rupture of the anterior cruciate ligament and/or damage to the collateral ligaments. In a few cases the torn part of the meniscus is dislocated between the condyles, causing a locking of the joint with accompanying pain. In most cases there is pain, swelling and a possible 'clicking' in the joint line with flexion and extension. Damage to the medial meniscus may also occur through its connection with the medial collateral ligament. Clinical diagnosis is difficult, but an arthroscope (a small instrument which can be used to visualise a joint and to perform small surgical repairs) may be able to locate and correct the problem by removing the free flap of damaged meniscus through the arthroscope.

- Anterior knee pain is very common in the growing dancer. This may be caused by a patello-femoral dysfunction or malalignment, or overuse. It often occurs as a consequence of a past injury.

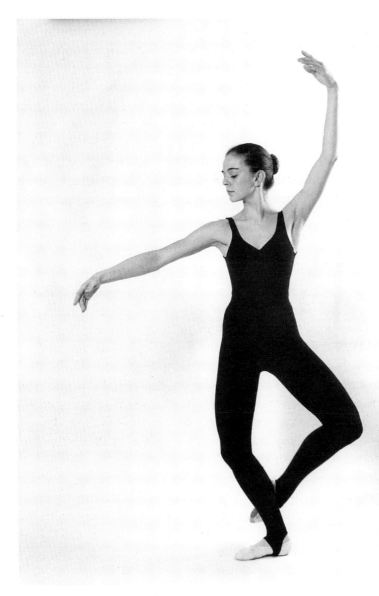

Plate 11. The knee en fondu.

- Dislocation of the patella may result from an instability around the ligaments of the patella. Sometimes in growing children the patellar ligament may be abnormally long and the patella abnormally small. This may mean that the patella moves in a lateral direction when the knee is extended. People who tend to have recurrent dislocation may need to have a surgical repair.
- Osteochondritis dissecans causes pain in the knee and is sometimes found in the growing dancer. The condition is caused by a free-floating body in the knee joint, usually a piece of joint cartilage with a thin layer of bone from the epiphysis. This starts with a local bone death (necrosis) below the epiphyseal plate and is mostly found by the medial femoral condyle.
- 'Jumper's knee' is damage to the patellar ligament (the tendon of the quadriceps muscle) often caused by large jumps, or faulty landings. It is most common in men. Pain is felt by the lower end of the patella on the tendon before it inserts into the tibia. Sometimes a tear occurs in the tendon which may need surgical repair.
- Instability of the knee may be caused by rupture of some of the supporting ligaments of the knee. When the knee is extended there is no sideways instability because of tension in the cruciate ligaments. However, when the knee is flexed to 15–20 degrees, the ligaments are relaxed and there is often a sideways instability. If one of the collateral ligaments is damaged there may be evident looseness or subluxation (partial dislocation) of the patella.
- Trauma to the knee such as a fall or repeated weight bearing on the knee may cause a bursitis, an inflammation of any of the many bursae in the knee. Swelling and pain often very local to the damaged area will be found.

*   *   *

The knee joint transmits the body weight from the large femur downwards to the smaller tibia. In dancers the shins are susceptible to much stress, so good alignment of the knees is vital for the efficient muscle action in the lower leg.

The leg

The tibia is the main weight-bearing bone in the lower leg. The proximal and distal ends of the tibia articulate with the fibula. There is a strong membrane between the two bones called the interosseous membrane. The fibula is a thin bone which runs parallel to the tibia. The inferior (lower) end of the tibia finishes in a large bony prominence called the medial malleolus, more commonly called the ankle bone. The inferior end of the fibula finishes in a bony prominence called the lateral malleolus. These two malleoli form the mortice for the ankle joint (Fig. 15).

Muscles of the lower leg

There are three muscle groups in the calf: the muscles at the front of the shin responsible for flexing the foot (dorsiflexion); those at the back of the calf responsible for pointing the foot (plantar flexion); and those at the lateral side of the calf responsible for inversion and eversion of the foot.

- The muscles at the front of the tibia are extensor muscles. The biggest is the tibialis anterior. This arises at the lateral side of the tibia and passes in front of the ankle to insert into the base of the first metatarsal. Its tendon is visible in dorsiflexion of the ankle. Other extensors of the lower leg are the toe extensors: extensors digitorum longus and brevis (which go to the second, third, fourth, fifth toes and pulls them upwards towards the body), and the extensors hallucis longus and brevis (which go to the first toe and pulls the toe upwards). Both toe extensors also extend the foot at the ankle (dancers refer to this as flexing the foot). These anterior calf muscles have strong retinaculae to keep the tendons from bowing upwards (Fig. 16).
- The posterior calf muscles are the gastrocnemius, a fleshy superficial muscle, and the deeper soleus muscle. These two muscles unite to form a common tendon, the Achilles tendon, which inserts into the calcaneus. The gastrocnemius arises from two origins above the knee at the back of the femur; therefore this muscle acts over two joints, the knee and the ankle. The gastrocnemius is very active in walking in the propulsive phrase of moving forwards. The soleus originates from the back of the tibia and fibula. As it inserts below the knee it can plantar flex the foot when the knee is bent. It is also an important postural

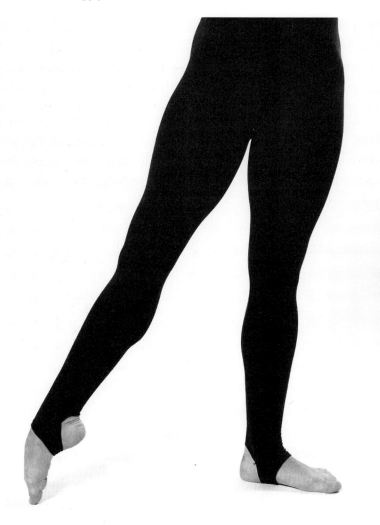

Plate 12. The leg (foot in plantar flexion).

muscle. The action of these two muscles is to plantar flex (point) the foot, although the gastrocnemius can also flex the knee.

- Deep to the soleus muscles are the tibialis posterior and the long flexor muscles: the flexor digitorum longus (which goes to the second, third, fourth, and fifth toes to point them), and the flexor hallucis longus (which goes to the big toe to point it). The tibialis posterior also plantar flexes the foot, and in the standing position it supports the arch of the foot. The tendons of these last three muscles pass behind and below the medial malleolus (ankle bone) and are situated inside tendon sheaths (Fig. 17).

- The muscles at the side of the calf are the peroneal muscles. The

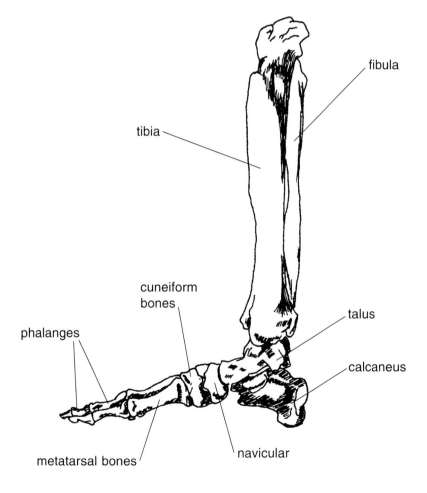

Fig. 15. The right lower leg and foot viewed from the medial aspect.

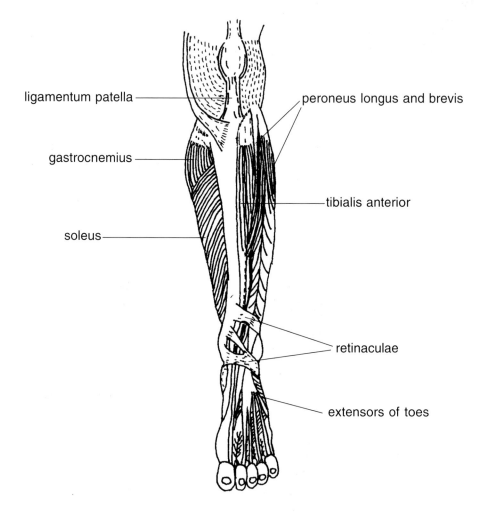

ligamentum patella

peroneus longus and brevis

gastrocnemius

tibialis anterior

soleus

retinaculae

extensors of toes

Fig. 16. The left knee and lower leg showing anterior calf muscles and toe extensors.

peroneus longus and brevis arise from the fibula and run down to the back of the lateral malleolus to run along the foot. The peroneus brevis inserts into the base of the fifth metatarsal, and the longus crosses underneath the foot to insert into the first metatarsal. They act as evertors of the foot (sickling outwards), and the peroneus longus can act as a dorsiflexor. They are important for the dancer when on pointe to maintain the integrity of the alignment of the calf, ankle and foot.

*   *   *

The tibia transmits the weight of the body down to the ankle joint. A wide range of movement can be made with the foot, because many muscles that act on the foot originate in the calf. The alignment of the tibia and the foot is critical to the integrity of the ankle and foot.

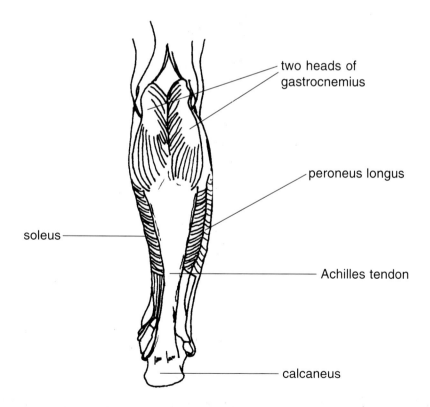

Fig. 17. The right posterior calf muscles.

The ankle and foot

The bones of the ankle and foot are:
- The distal ends of the tibia and fibula
- The talus
- The calcaneus
- The navicular
- The cuboid
- The first, second, third cuneiforms
- The 5 metatarsals
- The 14 phalanges
- The 2 sesamoid bones

The ankle joint is formed between the ends of the tibia and the fibula and the talus bone of the foot. It is a synovial hinge joint capable of flexion and extension. However, movement is not purely horizontal, as its axis is turned out to about 15 degrees. The two malleoli bones (ends of tibia and fibula) extend below the talus, forming a saddle type joint. All articular surfaces are covered in hyaline cartilage. The joint capsule is lax at the front and back, but fairly tight at the sides of the joint.

The subtalar joint is formed by the talus articulating with the calcaneus and by the talo-calcaneo-navicular bones articulating with each other. This joint has an axis in an oblique direction. Inversion and eversion occur at this joint. Inversion is when the sole of the foot faces inwards (also called supination), eversion when the sole of the foot is 'fished' outwards (also called pronation). The subtalar is a complex joint surrounded by its own weak capsular ligament.

The en pointe position is a combination of plantar flexion and inversion in the hindfoot. In the deep plié position the dorsiflexion of the ankle is supplemented with an eversion in the hindfoot.

Bones of the foot

There are three groups of bones in the foot: the bones of the tarsus, those of the metatarsals, and the phalanges (Fig. 18).
- The talus articulates with the tibia and fibula. It transfers the weight of the body forwards to the toes and backwards to the heel. At the back of the talus there is a flat prominence called the posterior pro-

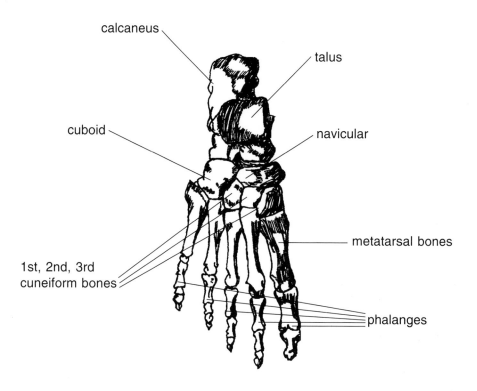

Fig. 18. The right foot viewed from above.

cess. On this process a small separate bone can sometimes develop (in about 8–13% of dancers) called the os trigonum.

- The calcaneus, commonly called the heel bone, is the largest bone in the foot. The sustentaculum tali is a prominent projection on the calcaneus. The Achilles tendon is attached to the posterior surface of the calcaneus.
- The navicular bone is on the medial aspect of the foot. It has a tuberosity which may be felt though the skin. It articulates posteriorly with the talus, laterally with the cuneiform bones, and anteriorly with the metatarsals.

- The three cuneiform bones – medial, intermediate and lateral – articulate with the metatarsal bones.
- The cuboid bone, so called due to its square shape, is on the lateral side of the foot, situated between the calcaneus and the fourth and fifth metatarsal bones.
- The metatarsus, with five metatarsal bones, each leading to a toe, forms the shaft of the forefoot. The bases of the metatarsal bones articulate with the tarsal bones, the heads articulate with the phalanges (toes). The base of the fifth metatarsal is often prominent and may be felt through the skin.
- The two small sesamoid bones (so called because they are a similar in shape to a sesame seed) are situated in between the heads of the first and second metatarsals. They are not always completely ossified and can be formed of tough fibrous tissue. The actual function of the sesamoid bones in the foot is not well documented.
- The phalanges correspond to the digits of the fingers; there are two to the great toe and three to each of the other toes. The joint between the metatarsals and phalanges is called the metatarsophalangeal joint.

Ligaments

- On the medial side of the ankle joint is the deltoid ligament, which runs from the medial malleolus and fans outwards to the talus, navicular and a bony prominence on the calcaneum called the sustentaculum tali.
- The tibia and fibula are kept together by the anterior and posterior tibiofibular ligaments. The latter is very strong.
- Between the navicular and sustentaculum tali is the spring ligament.
- At the back of the ankle is the very strong talofibular ligament.
- In the deepest layer of the sole of the foot is a very strong ligament called the long ligament, which runs from the lower side of the calcaneus to the tarsus and metatarsal bones.

In the sole of the foot below the skin is a very thick triangular fibrous structure from the front of the heel to the metatarsophalangeal joints (toe joints). This is called the plantar fascia. When the toes are bent upwards it can felt as a hard cord.

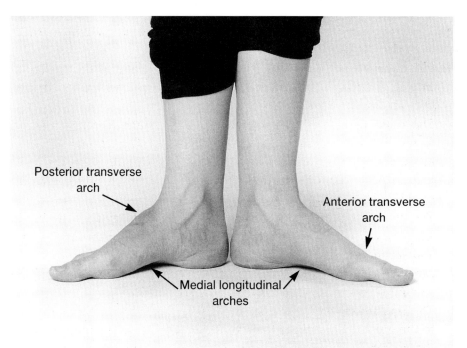

Plate 13. The arches of the foot.

The arches of the foot

There are four arches of the foot (Plates 13 & 14):

- The anterior transverse arch runs across the metatarsophalangeal joints.
- The posterior transverse arch runs across the highest part of the foot, by the talus.
- The medial longitudinal arch runs down from the calcaneus, through the navicular, and three cuneiform bones into the medial three metatarsals. This is a fairly high arch.
- The lateral longitudinal arch runs down the lateral side of the foot from the calcaneus, through the cuboid and then through the lateral two metatarsals.

The arches provide a dynamic platform for the foot and together form a

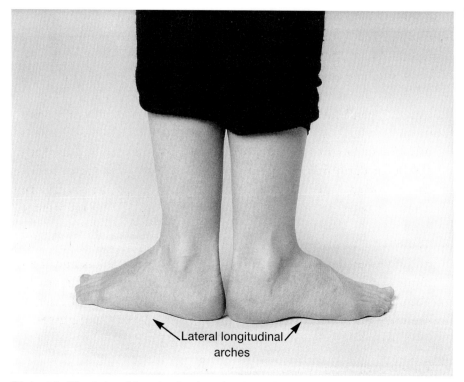

Plate 14. The lateral longitudinal arch of the foot.

dome shape which gives the foot resilience, the ability to absorb shock from impact, and a firm base for support. The design of the arches of the foot gives the foot tremendous strength, especially important for the dancer. They are able to balance the weight of the body on a tiny platform when on pointe or demi-pointe, and to withstand the increased weight of the body as it descends from a jump, often on one leg. The arches are supported by the shape of the bones themselves, and by strong ligaments and tendons acting like a sling to maintain the arches. However, due to misuse or abuse, these ligaments may be overstretched and the strength of the arch may be diminished. The medial longitudinal arch tends to be most susceptible to injury if the dancer places the weight incorrectly on the inside of the foot. Constant pronation will cause the medial arch to fail.

'Flat foot' is a congenital condition (present at birth) and exhibits a very reduced medial arch. This type of foot is not suitable for vocational dance training, as little can be done to alter the shape of the arch.

Muscles of the foot and ankle

Some of the muscles that act on the foot and ankle have already been considered in the discussion of calf muscles. The muscles of the foot and ankle mostly originate in the calf and act upon the foot via their tendons in order for the foot to be streamlined, not thick with muscle. There are, however, several layers of small muscles acting on the foot. Some of these are:

- Muscles in the sole of the foot, including the flexor hallucis brevis, the flexor digiti minimi, the adductor hallucis, the abductor hallucis, the abductor digiti minimi, and the flexor digitorum accessorius. These muscles act to give the foot a wide range of movement options.
- The lumbricals and interossei muscles. These small muscles around and between the metatarsal bones and phalanges can extend the toe joints and control flexion of the metatarsophalangeal joints, and can abduct and adduct the toes. They are important for the dancer, and their use is improved with strong battements tendus and glissés.

Common problems of the foot and ankle

- The os trigonum (sometimes formed at the back of the talus) may cause problems for a dancer. When a relevé is performed, the abnormally long process may irritate the back of the ankle, as the bone is pressed into the synovial capsule of the ankle joint. This is accompanied by pain and swelling felt at the front of the joint.
- Dorsiflexion of the foot is halted when the talus bone contacts the tibia. Forced dorsiflexion may encourage the development of a small bone spur, or exostosis, at the upper edge of the talus. The same problem of a bone spur may also occur at the back of the calcaneus and cause pain when the foot is pointed. Dancers often prefer to wear shoes that are a very snug fit, and this can encourage excessive wear at the back of the calcaneus. If such an exostosis does occur, it may have to be surgically removed (Plate 15).
- A sprain of the ankle may occur after a fall off pointe resulting in a sudden inversion of the foot. In some cases the sprain is so severe that all the surrounding ligaments are ruptured; the joint capsule may also be ruptured. In such cases there is an abnormal looseness in the joint and local symptoms of pain and swelling around the lateral malleolus.

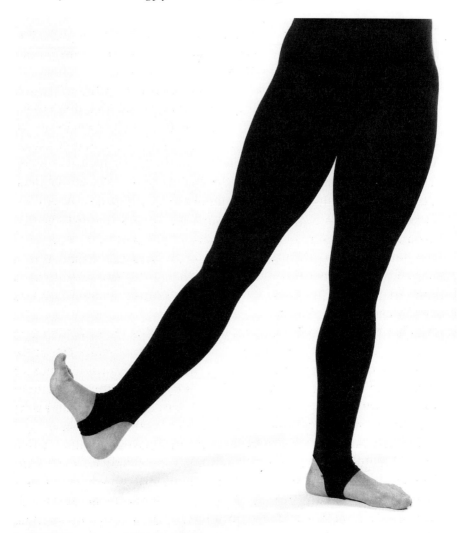

Plate 15. The foot in dorsiflexion.

There are varying degrees of ankle sprain, and it is important to ascertain if ligaments have been ruptured. It is quite rare for the sprain to be on the inside of the ankle.

- Occasionally there may be abnormal bone growth in the metatarsal head in children. This is called Freiberg's disease, and results in a flattened head of a metatarsal, possibly with some osteoarthrosis. The dancer has pain when going on demi-pointe and there may be swelling and tenderness around the joint.

- The first metatarsophalangeal joint may be deformed with lateral displacement of the toe. This deformity is called hallux valgus (or bunion). It is unfortunately very common amongst dancers. The first metatarsal head is pressed against the upper part of a shoe, with resultant thickening of the skin around the area and irritation of a prominent bursa. The increased bone growth is the body's response to constant pressure. In severe cases of hallux valgus the sesamoid bones are dislocated laterally.

- Another problem of the first toe is hallux rigidus. This is a stiff first toe joint with limited movement and pain, and possibly osteoarthrosis. The big toe is very important for the dancer for push-off, and for mobility to point. Hallux rigidus may be operated upon successfully for ordinary people, but for dancers it is not often successful, as the mobility necessary for a dancer in this joint is rarely recovered.

- The tendon sheath of the three muscles that pass below the medial malleolus (tibialis posterior, flexor digitorum longus and flexor hallucis longus) may cause problems. The tendon sheath acts as protection for the tendons, but occasionally can become inflamed through overuse. This is called peritendinitis. There may be pain and swelling in the local area, exacerbated by movement.

- Although their function is not well known, the sesamoid bones in the foot may cause a problem for dancers, as they are situated in a position which receives much stress. Tap dancers in particular may suffer from a fractured sesamoid bone, or an inflammation of the bursa between the two bones. Repeated stress to the area under the first and second metatarsophalangeal joints may cause, or at least exacerbate the problem.

- A painful condition around the heads of the metatarsals caused by degeneration of the bone may cause pain usually associated with one of the first three metatarsal heads. This is called metatarsalgia. If damage is extended to the sensory nerves in the foot it is called Morton's neuroma. This is a nodule on the nerve, and may cause pain and tenderness with reduced sensitivity in the toes.

*   *   *

It is important to understand the anatomy of the body – the bones, joints, muscles, and structures. But it is equally important to understand how to apply that knowledge. The body structures have been discussed individually for clarity, but the interrelationships that exist in the musculo-skeletal system are many. In a dancer these relationships are refined, and critical to the development of training.

Part 3

The Dancer in Action

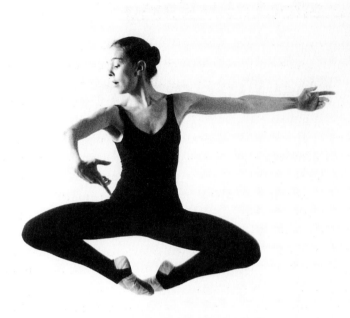

Plate 16. The dancer in action.

The effect of training

We learn by repetition. When we first attempt a movement there is generally excessive muscle use and much tension in the body. This is easily demonstrated by the professional dancer, who makes a difficult movement appear easy because the body has learnt how to produce the movement efficiently, with as little tension as possible. By repetition of a movement the dancer learns to use the minimal amount of muscular contraction to reproduce the step required. By eliminating excessive tension in the body the pattern of a movement becomes ingrained in the body. It is easy to describe this as 'muscle memory'. There are complicated functions going on inside the body involving subcortical conditioning and neurological pathways that make an initially complicated series of actions become a smooth relaxed action. The dancer no longer has to tell each set of muscles in the body how to do a pas de chat; the 'muscle memory' already has that information.

This is important to remember when teaching a new step or a complicated enchaînement to younger dancers. The first few times the movement will appear clumsy and full of tension and strain. With repetition the movement becomes more fluid and easier to perform. Of course, not all students will be able to establish these pathways (similar to a short cut on a journey) at the same time. Some will require a longer period of time.

Beneficial stretching

As has previously been discussed, the dancer needs to stretch and work the muscles of the body repeatedly. With the demand for increasingly high extensions of the legs, it becomes more and more important to understand how to stretch the muscles in a way that is of real benefit to the dancer.

Types of stretching

- Ballistic stretches. These are the 'bouncy' stretches sometimes still performed by teachers and dancers in an effort to stretch muscles, usually the hamstrings. The student bounces forwards over the legs in a quick, sudden movement. This has some effect, but very minimal lasting effect. Modern dance training tends to use this type of stretch, as it is rhythmical, and easy to ask for 'eight stretches each way', for example. It is not, however, an effective way of stretching muscles, and may possibly do more harm than good, especially if combined with rotation and twisting in the spine. There may be microscopic tearing of muscle fibres when a sudden stretch is placed on a muscle. This type of stretching is inefficient as it elicits the 'stretch reflex', which initiates a contraction in the muscle when sudden stretch and tension is placed on it.
- Passive stretches, or long slow stretches. This is when a muscle is placed in a 'comfortable' stretch and held there, usually by the force of gravity, or assisted by gentle pressure. For example, the dancer sits with the legs straight out in front and relaxes over the knees to stretch the hamstrings. If a muscle is held in this position for a period of time (sources dispute exact length of time, but it is generally held to be several minutes) it will not activate the stretch reflex, as although some tension is placed on the muscle, it is gradual rather than sudden. Special sensors called the Golgi tendon organs, found where the muscle and tendon join together, are able to sense tension in a muscle when it is stretched slowly and at the end of the range. This sense can inhibit the contraction of a muscle and allow deep stretching to take place. This method of stretching has been shown to be more effective than ballistic type bouncing.

- Proprioceptive neuromuscular facilitation (PNF). This is a technique for stretching that allows the body to use its natural ability to lengthen a muscle after 'reciprocal' inhibition has been placed on a muscle. This means that after a group of muscles has been placed in a 'comfortable' stretch, a contraction is elicited in the muscle. This is achieved by meeting the force of the contraction with an opposing force (usually by a partner). After several seconds of this type of contraction (again, sources dispute how long the contraction needs to be held), the muscle will relax sufficiently to allow it to be put in a new lengthened position. The benefit of this type of stretch is that the muscle group gains strength as well as flexibility. This is particularly effective for hamstrings and adductor stretches. The assisting partner must be well briefed and only match the force of the muscular contraction and not exceed the pressure. This form of stretching has been shown to be much more effective than ballistic methods (Plates 17 & 18).

Recent publications advise that when doing PNF techniques the amount of extensibility gained can be further enhanced by two mechanisms: breathing and visualisation. Slow deep breathing as a stretch is increased can encourage the muscle to relax and therefore lengthen. Visualising the muscle lengthening and having a positive image of it can also, it is believed, have favourable effects on extending the length of a muscle. If students understand what is happening physiologically they are more able to visualise the fibres increasing in length (see R. Stephens in Solomon, Minton & Solomon, *Preventing Dance Injuries*, 1990, p. 284).

When to stretch

It is important to stretch muscles when they are warm and more pliable. The end of class is an excellent time to do some beneficial stretches, especially at the end of the range of movement. It may be appropriate to do some gentle stretches at the start of class, but even these should be done after a brief physical warm-up (jogging, skipping – anything to raise the heart rate and core temperature of the body). These pre-class stretches should be slow and gentle and not at the end of the normal range. Many dancers like to start class by sitting in a stretched position, but this probably does little for them if the body is cold. Too many

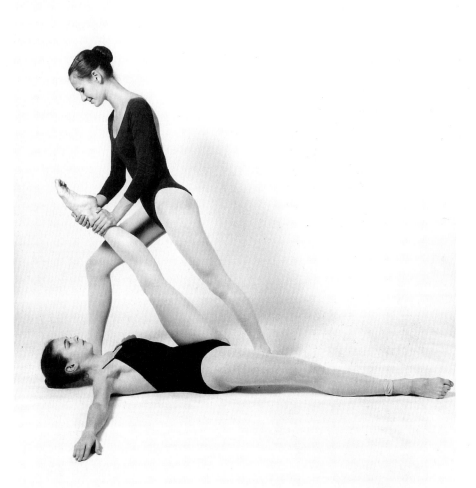

Plate 17. Proprioceptive neuromuscular facilitation (PNF) stretching technique, showing partner assisting by meeting the contraction of the hamstrings with an opposing force.

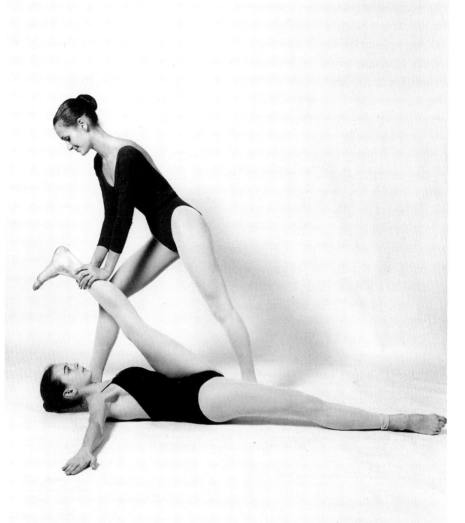

Plate 18. The leg is then able to stretch further and repeat the exercise in the new lengthened position.

stretches at the start of the class will merely allow the body to cool down further from relative inactivity.

During the normal class more specific stretches can be progressively incorporated into the exercises as the body warms up. These exercises should be appropriate to the age and standard of the participants, and the demands of training.

Factors affecting flexibility

- Age. Young children are fairly flexible. They may start to become less flexible as they reach the age of about 10 or 11. Flexibility may then improve throughout adolescence, although it will rarely reach the facility of early childhood.
- Gender. Females appear to be more flexible than males at all ages.
- Activity. The more active a person is, the more likely he or she is to retain flexibility. This flexibility may diminish if a period of inactivity occurs, as may happen during a long holiday, and it may take a while to recover.
- Joint mobility. Flexibility in joints will be governed by the soft tissues surrounding that joint. For example, if the ligaments and joint capsules are lax and give a wide range of movement, the joint will be able to move freely. The hypermobile body (usually congenitally predetermined), although seen to be aesthetically desirable, is prone to injury and must be very carefully trained. Sufficient strength to control movement is vital.
- Tension. If an individual tends to hold a lot of tension in the body, flexibility may be affected as the 'release' threshold of the muscle groups will be higher. This means that in a habitually tense dancer, flexibility may be reduced unless specific countermeasures are taken.

Warming up and warming down

It cannot be overstressed how important a thorough warm-up is. It prepares the mind and body for class; it is vital in terms of injury prevention and correct muscular use. If a proper warm-up routine is done before class, the dancer will be able to move more effectively at the beginning of class, be less likely to sustain damage, and be able to endure more throughout the performance.

Warming up increases the body temperature so that nerve impulses can travel more quickly. It is very difficult to execute rapid movements when the body is cold. A good warm-up should:
- Raise the body temperature.
- Raise the heart rate and blood circulation of the body. Blood is important in bringing oxygen to muscle tissues: nutrition is stored in the blood and waste products from the working muscle are contained in blood.
- Stretch the large muscle groups and warm up the joints. As the core temperature of the body rises, the extensibility (the ability to stretch) of muscles improves. A warm environment allows for a faster transmission of nerve impulses, and faster speed of muscle contraction.
- Improve the viscosity of synovial fluid, encouraging smoother joint action.

Raising the body temperature can only be done by actually working the body. Dancers like to think that wearing lots of baggy layers and sitting in front of the radiator constitutes a good warm-up! Actually getting out of breath in the warm-up is important, as this will stimulate the body to increase the heart rate and respiration rate. A few laps of jogging around the studio would not be inappropriate.

Any excessive forms of stretching or bouncing can result in muscle or tendon injuries, and should be avoided. A slow, gentle, methodical warm-up is far better. This should be done to stretch main muscles in order to get them ready for fast and effective contraction, reduce any shortening of muscles that has occurred, and prepare the heart and lungs for action.

Having stretched the large muscles of the body and gently mobilised the major joints, each dancer can focus on an area that is of particular importance to him or her personally. For example, a dancer with short calf muscles and tight Achilles tendons should spend time stretching out the calf muscles slowly and gently. It could be a good habit for dancers to do a general warm-up followed by a personal warm-up specific to their own physiques.

After about 10–15 minutes the dancer will be physically and mentally more alert and ready for action. This warm-up time is also important in terms of mental preparation and the ability to 'focus' on internal messages from the body. It is learning time for the dancer to get to know the body and understand how best to work it. In this way dancers learn to take personal responsibility for their individual physiques.

We are only beginning to understand the importance of warming down. After a long class when the body has been working hard, and is probably at maximum cardiac output with a high temperature and pulse rate, it is more beneficial to wind down slowly than to stop working completely.

Working muscles produce a waste product called lactic acid. In the presence of sufficient oxygen the body is able to recycle this into glycogen, a muscle fuel. An excess of lactic acid can cause muscle cramps and aching muscles. So by working the body gently and encouraging good breathing techniques the lactic acid is given a chance to combine with oxygen and reused. Warming down also allows the heart rate a chance to slow down and the temperature to drop slowly so it calms the dancer. A sudden change from an extreme state of activity into complete rest does not give the body a chance to readjust itself. A gradual slowing down of output while doing some gentle activity is ideal.

A good warm-down combined with gentle stretches can help the dancer avoid delayed onset muscle soreness (DOMS). This can occur 24 to 48 hours after unusually vigorous muscle action, and causes discomfort and pain. For a well-trained dancer used to performing exercises appropriate to demands, DOMS may be rare. However, for a dancer returning to class after a rest or rehabilitation, or a dancer working in a style or technique that is unfamiliar, DOMS can cause problems. This may be avoided to some extent by being sufficiently aware of the problem, and doing slow, careful post-exercise stretches. (Teachers and dancers often suffer from very sore calves on return to class after a long break. This may be a form of DOMS, and is very painful!)

Many teachers will not have time in a normal dance lesson to spend class time doing a thorough warm-up and warm-down. Perhaps a couple of times a month they could teach the dancers what to do and how to do the exercises (including explaining the physiological importance of this) and then leave the dancers with the responsibility of coming to class already partially warmed up.

Breathing

The mechanism of breathing has not been discussed at length, as this is not a physiology textbook. However, it is important for teachers to understand basic breathing patterns for dancers.

We breathe by means of two mechanisms: the contraction of the intercostal muscles, which swing the rib cage upwards and outwards, and the contraction of the diaphragm muscle, which enlarges the thoracic cavity.

At the front of the body, the ribs are moved by intercostal muscles, with the diaphragm as an additional respiratory muscle. The dome-shaped diaphragm separates the thoracic cavity from the abdominal cavity and contracts downwards. In conjunction with the intercostal muscles, the thoracic cavity is increased and air is inspired through the lungs. The diaphragm then relaxes back to its dome-shaped position.

There are three types of breathing:

- Apical breathing takes place at the top of the lungs and rib cage. Little air is taken in during apical breathing, and as it can involve use of the shoulders and neck, it is not aesthetically pleasing, and creates much tension in the upper thorax.
- Diaphragmatic breathing focuses on deep breaths concentrated in the lower part of the thorax. It is often called abdominal breathing, as the stomach is relaxed and extends outwards during inspiration. Again, this is not aesthetically pleasing for the dancer.
- Lateral breathing engages the intercostal muscles to expand the rib cage. The diaphragm is held fairly still so the line of the body remains calm. It is called lateral breathing because the action takes place mostly sideways in the ribs. This method fills the lower lobes of the lungs and is very efficient. This is the form of breathing most used by dancers during slow, sustained movements.

In fast-paced enchaînements, all forms of breathing are used to supply the body with sufficient oxygen. Additional muscles in the shoulders, neck and abdomen are recruited to aid rapid respiration and give the body extra oxygen.

If muscles have a sufficient supply of oxygen they are able to reconvert lactic acid, a waste product of a working muscle, into an energy source for recycling. However, if excessive muscular contraction is required with insufficient oxygen, lactic acid can accumulate, causing aching and cramps – a good reason to make sure dancers breathe properly and have sufficient 'recovery' time.

Good breathing technique can aid the proper execution of dance movements, add dynamics, and add a pleasing quality to port de bras. Some steps may be enhanced by a specific breathing pattern, for example breathing out as a pirouette is performed, breathing in during a rise, and remembering to breathe during adage.

Most dance classes tend to be anaerobic in nature towards the end of the lesson. Aerobic exercise means that the output of energy is balanced by the amount of oxygen in the body, so activity can continue for a period of time. Anaerobic exercise means that for a short period of time the amount of muscle action required to produce a movement is not met by the amount of oxygen in the body. Muscles can work without sufficient levels of oxygen in the body for a short time but the body must then replace the oxygen as soon as possible with deep, rapid breathing.

Dancers are not generally known for their aerobic fitness. The ability to sustain a long role or performance is usually developed during the rehearsal process, not in the class. Perhaps this is an aspect of general fitness training that needs to be looked at. Appropriate levels of aerobic fitness training could be included at some time during preparation for a performance, or more ideally, as an everyday part of class.

Balance

The ability to balance comes from a combination of many messages received by the brain. Most information comes from inside the ear, where there are three semicircular canals. The canals lie in three dimensions and can therefore detect all movement through a combination of messages from all three. The canals are filled with fluid; tiny hairs sense the movement of the fluid when the head or body is tilted. Added to the information received from the ear, the brain receives information from the eyes and from sensory receptors and proprioceptors in the soles of the feet (Plate 19).

A body can balance when the centre line of gravity is placed over the base of support. The larger the base of support, the easier it is to balance. For example, it is easier to balance when standing in second position than when standing on one leg on demi-pointe. It is possible to balance in asymmetrical positions and move the centre of gravity (as in much contemporary dance). The dancer uses 'kinaesthetic awareness' (an understanding of the position of the body) to aid the balance process. This 'muscle' sense can be best demonstrated at the ankle when balancing on one leg: the muscles around the ankle may make tiny adjustments and contractions to improve the placement of the foot. This happens not through voluntary control but through the kinaesthetic sense.

For the growing student the act of balancing is made even harder as the body changes in mass and length for several years. If a student is finding it particularly difficult to find balance, it is possible to enhance some of the messages sent to the brain by taking the ballet shoes off and finding the balance with bare feet. This will give the sensory receptors in the soles of the foot more opportunity to receive information.

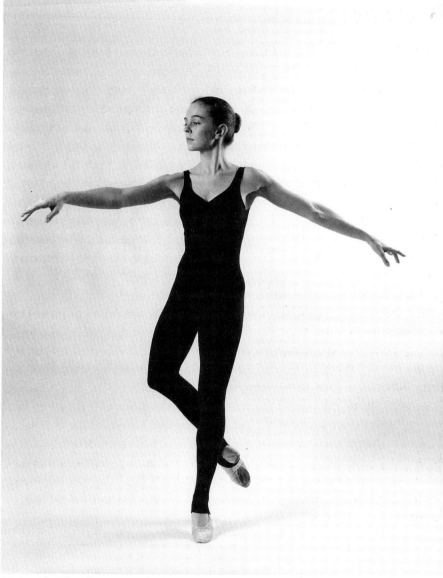

Plate 19. The dancer on balance.

Muscle balance

A different form of 'balance' is muscular balance – the relationship between two antagonistic muscle groups, or the recruitment of muscle groups to perform an action. A dancer's training tends to produce one set of muscles that are overused, leaving another set of muscles underused. For example, the lateral rotator muscles are used a lot in classical training, yet the medial rotator muscles are hardly used. The typical picture that this presents is bulky buttock muscles, with reduced mobility in the hip socket due to lack of strength in the medial rotators and understretched lateral rotators. These, in turn, could cause the iliotibial band running down the outer thigh to become very tight, and may cause the patella to be pulled laterally away from its natural groove. This example is only seen in the worst cases, but any muscular imbalance leaves the dancer predisposed to injury.

Simple actions such as stretching the lateral rotators and occasionally using the medial rotators, stretching the overused plantar flexors (to point the foot), and working the dorsiflexors (to pull the foot upwards), can help avoid the imbalance syndrome.

It may be necessary to reassess how dancers' training is biomechanically structured in order to prevent overworked/underused muscles.

The growth spurt

It is not within the premise of this book to give any psychological insights into a dancer's training. However, an understanding of some of the physical changes that occur in training may explain why some students may have a poor self-image during adolescence. The following is common-sense advice from many years of experience, not from any training in psychology.

From the ages of about 13–16 for a girl and about 14–17 for a boy, the growth spurt occurs. This is a time of rapid increase in height and weight. Bones grow faster than muscles, so there will be several times when students may outgrow their own strength. Suddenly the dance student will be unable to do exercises that were once easy to perform. Typical examples of this are balancing exercises, pirouettes, adage and controlled extensions, and allegro. The long bones of the body are not yet surrounded by sufficiently strong musculature, and once simple tasks now become awkward and difficult. The timing of the growth spurt often coincides with great hormonal changes in the body, peer group pressure, and the development from child to young adult. For the girl there are very obvious physical changes to buttocks and breasts. In this situation, being in a leotard surrounded by mirrors is probably the last place a dance student wants to be.

Although it may seem a very obvious statement, it is vitally important to reassure teenage dancers that when the growth spurt slows down they will recover strength and technique. The knowledge that it is normal to be unable to control the body fully during growth, and that with time and strength the body will emerge as a very capable and skilled instrument, will encourage adolescent dance students. Much frustration can be avoided by knowledge and understanding of the physical changes.

The growth spurt may be over in one year, or in three to four years. For the majority of that time normal classes can be done. For those students who return from a holiday noticeably taller, some modification of class work may be necessary. The knee is particularly vulnerable at this time.

This is perhaps a time for the teacher to initiate alternative strengthening exercises at the end of class instead of repeating an enchaînement. These may include exercises for strengthening the torso (especially the abdominal muscles), the hamstrings, and quadriceps muscle groups. It is also a time when much encouragement needs to be given to the student, as the teenage ego is so very fragile. If the students can recognise that their teacher is aware and understands their physical changes they will feel more comfortable in themselves. All too often a damaging attitude to the body can develop during this time as students continually compare themselves to others – a potentially harmful practice. The more a dance student can understand the body, take responsibility for strengthening it and following an agreed programme of exercises, the more positive his or her self-image will be.

It may be during the growth spurt that serious decisions are made about future careers and full-time training. Encouraging students to be realistic is always a difficult task – some are too full of self-doubt, others too full of unrealistic dreams. The teachers or mentors that students come to for guidance need a good understanding of physical, psychological and emotional development of the dance student.

There are many excellent books on the psychology of the performer and sports psychology that are very appropriate for the dancer and dance teacher.

Conclusion

Having studied and learnt about the body from the inside out, the teacher may use this knowledge in the dance studio. The dancer may understand the 'how' and the 'why' of the body, and take personal responsibility for it. Choreographers may have respect for the delicate structures that are the building tools of their art. The artistic director may encourage dancers to work to their maximum, but not beyond it.

Whatever your personal reasons for wanting to learn about the anatomy of a dancer, you may be faced with choices. Knowledge brings change. An understanding of the body may change how you work from now on. You may of course decide that nothing needs to change in your daily class, but at least you will be making a choice based on knowledge, not assumptions. The science of anatomy and kinesiology empowers these choices. You have a right to make your own contribution to your own class. The dance art form that we all love will benefit.

The science and the art of dance has been nowhere better explained or discussed than in *Dance Kinesiology*, by Sally Sevey Fitt, and is a suitable conclusion to this book:

"Dance is an expressive art form that totally relies on human movement for communication. Choreography and performance are the two primary avenues of expression in dance . . . each of these two roles is potentially benefited by accurate scientific knowledge of human motion."

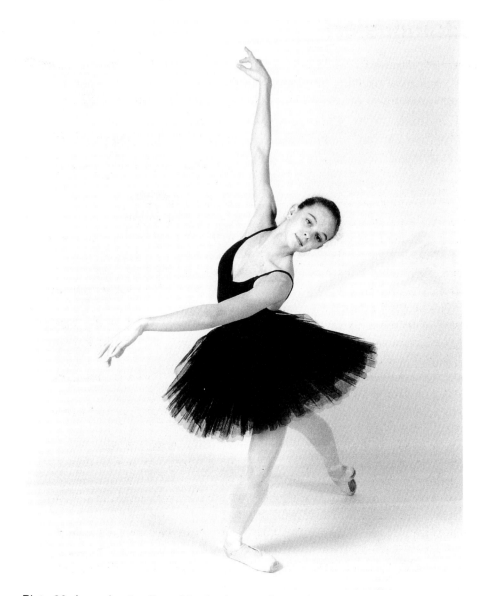

Plate 20. An understanding of the body may change how you move from now on.

Bibliography

Berardi, G. *Finding Balance: Fitness and Training for a Lifetime in Dance*, (Pennington, NJ: Princeton Book Co., 1991)

Brukner, P. & Khan, K. *Clinical Sports Medicine* (Sydney, Australis: McGraw Hill, 1993)

Clarkson, P.M. & Skriner, M. (eds). *The Science of Dance Training* (Champaign, IL: Human Kinetics, 1988)

deVries, H. & Housh, T. *Physiology of Exercise*, 5th edn (Wisconsin: Brown & Benchmark, 1994)

Fitt, S. S. *Dance Kinesiology* (New York: MacMillan, 1988)

Gray, H., *Gray's Anatomy*, 35th edn (Edinburgh: Longmans, 1973)

Gray, J.A. *Dance Instruction: Science Applied to the Art of Movement* (Champaign, IL: Human Kinetics, 1989)

Greig, V. *Inside Ballet Technique* (London: Dance Books, 1994)

Moffat, D. & Mottram, R. *Anatomy and Physiology for Physiotherapists* 2nd edn (Oxford: Blackwell, 1987)

Mosby's Medical and Nursing Dictionary 2nd edn (Missouri: C.V. Mosby, 1986)

Nagrin, D. *How to Dance Forever. Surviving against the Odds* (New York: William Morrow, 1988)

Paskeva, A. *Both Sides of the Mirror. The Science and Art of Ballet* (Pennington, NJ: Princeton Book Co., 1992)

Ryan, A. & Stephens, R. *The Dancer's Complete Guide to Healthcare and a Long Career* (Chicago: Bonus Books, 1988)

Ryan, A. & Stephens R., *The Healthy Dancer* (London: Dance Books, 1987)

Scott, W.M., Nisonson N. & Nicholas, J. (eds). *Principles of Sports Medicine* (Baltimore, Williams & Wilkins, USA, 1984)

Solomon, R., Minton, S., & Solomon, J. (eds). *Preventing Dance Injuries* (Reston, VA: American Alliance for Health, 1990)

Sweigard, L. *Human Movement Potential: Its Ideokinetic Facilitation* (New York: Harper & Row, 1974)

Thompson, C. *Manual of Structural Kinesiology* (St Louis: Times Mirror/Mosby, 1989)

Wilson, K. *Anatomy and Physiology* (London: Churchill Livingston, 1990)

About the Authors

Professor Eivind Ingemann Thomasen (1908–1988)

Professor Thomasen obtained his degree in Medicine from the University of Aarhus, Denmark, in 1946, and became a Doctor of Medicine in 1948. He was consultant in charge of The Orthopaedic Hospital in Aarhus from 1952 until his retirement in 1978. He was Professor of Orthopaedic Surgery at the University of Aarhus from 1958 until 1978.

His main publications were 'Myotonia, Thomsen Disease' (1948) and 'Diseases and Injuries of Ballet Dancers' (1982). He was a corresponding member of the American Orthopaedic Association and the British Orthopaedic Association, and Honourable Member of the Société Français d'Orthopédie et Traumatologie and the Nordic Orthopaedic Association.

Professor Thomasen married Helga Jansen in 1936 and they had three daughters. He died in 1988.

Rachel-Anne Rist

Rachel-Anne Rist is Head of Dance at the Arts Educational School, Tring, Hertfordshire. She is author of the book *The Injured Dancer* and of many articles on training techniques and dance medicine for dance and sports journals.

She is an Executive Committee member for the Royal Academy of Dancing, and UK Correspondent and Board member for the International Association of Dance Medicine and Science.

She has a masters degree in performing arts, and is currently involved in research on dance training.